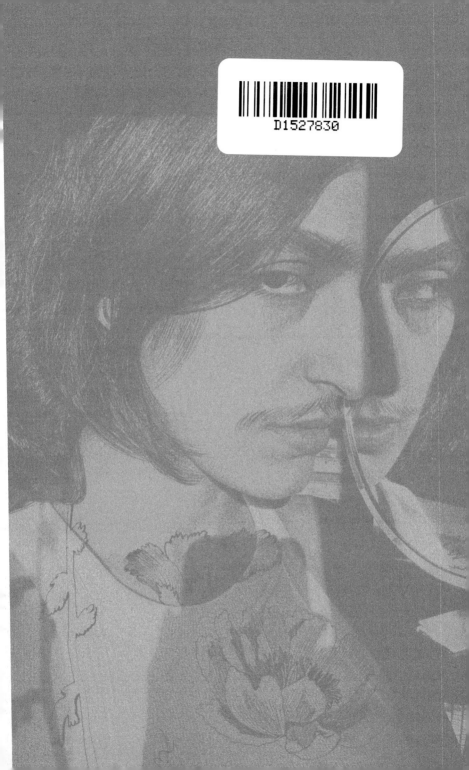

UGLINESS

MOSHTARI HILAL

Translated from the German by Elisabeth Lauffer

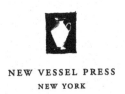

NEW VESSEL PRESS
NEW YORK

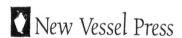

New Vessel Press

www.newvesselpress.com

Copyright © 2023 Carl Hanser Verlag GmbH & Co. KG, München
Translation copyright © 2025 Elisabeth Lauffer

The translation of this work was supported by a grant from the Goethe-Institut.

Library of Congress Cataloging-in-Publication Data
Hilal, Moshtari
[Hässlichkeit, English]
Ugliness/Moshtari Hilal; translation by Elisabeth Lauffer.
p. cm.
ISBN 978-1-954404-28-1
Library of Congress Control Number 2024938163
I. Germany—Nonfiction

This is a book about images. The images in our heads, on our faces, behind our eyes, on our tongues. It is also a book about gaze—the way we look at things and the way others absorb that gaze, and the way these looks become part of our bodies. This book is about seeing and being seen. This book is about the hatred (*Hass*) in ugliness (*Hässlichkeit*) and about the outer limit and opposite of beauty. It begins with me and ends in us all.

CONTENTS

I. HATRED

Hey, horseface,
where do you get off
using my face to
grin so sweetly?

That's not what I looked like
brushing my hair that morning.
That wasn't me.

I had laid out my clothes the night before,
color-coordinated,
with a practiced expression
and shy mouth.

Where do you get off
using my face to
grin so sweetly?

Now, give us a smile.
The photographer at our school
summons my smile.
Give us a smile,
and I smiled.

Where do you get off
using my face to
grin so sweetly?

I remembered the first YouTube comment
I ever got, the comment
that made me delete my first video:

Hey, horseface.

Where do you get off
using my face to
grin so sweetly?

I saw myself
in fourteen passport-photo-sized rectangles
and they gazed back.

It was exactly as A. had spelled it out for me in the school
hallway:

crooked teeth,
long face,
big nose.

At fourteen I learned fourteen times over
that I'm ugly.

Fourteen someones making a face in my place
on the sheet of photos in my mother's hand.

Was my smile
a distortion, or did it
leave me exposed?

We're not keeping these, I told my mother.
I don't need this picture, and I never
want to see it again. And I never
want this picture to see me.
My mother closed the envelope
that held my fourteen
grimacing faces.
She placed it folded up in her dresser:
　　　　That's my darling daughter.

An ugly child only a mother could love.

I dig up that photo for this book.
I search in vain
for an ugly horseface.
All I find is the picture of a child
flashing her teeth,
smiling for what will be the last time
in fourteen years.

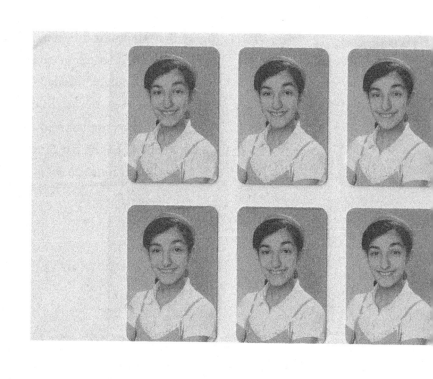

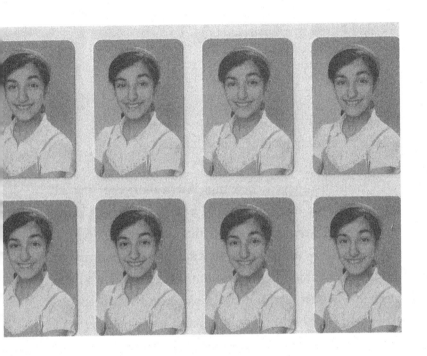

SELF-PORTRAIT

As a kid I drew in a small notebook

what I would be when I grew up.

I drew a woman.
I drew a woman with long, smooth legs.

On the first page I drew myself in a short skirt and silk blouse with my hair up. I would become a lawyer like the lawyers on American TV shows that aired at 8:15 p.m. in our living room, the lawyers who strode through courtrooms, around Manhattan, and across our TV screen. I would be attractive, attract attention and hold gazes, turn heads as I passed. In high heels, my long smooth legs would carry me about, women and men alike stealing glances. Their looks would pool at my feet, where I'd trap them with my red soles, gliding untouched through the crowd, dodging no one, not a shoulder refusing to make way for mine, not an unrequited smile.

My feet four inches from the floor,
my nose five feet, six inches from the floor.
If I'm remembering correctly, I don't remember any nose.

I shaped my face in the shape of a heart
atop a body like an hourglass
with eyes like almonds and lips like pillows soft as velvet.
My smooth legs would evoke the shiny glass facades
of the Twin Towers; my smooth hair would resemble oil.

I drew a woman, the woman I would be,
who would show her white teeth when she smiled
and brush her silky hair
out of her delicate face
with her fine, manicured fingers
and cross her smooth, clean, delicate,
silky, sleek legs.

She was right there before my eyes; I knew every last inch
of this woman's body. In my head I practiced wearing her body
like an alien skin that was meant to be mine. A skin I was copy-
ing off someone else. I observed what defined the beautiful and
successful women whose ranks I wished to join and did not
include my mother and aunts. I would be different from them
by choice. I would be a woman who knew what she wanted.

At age fourteen I bought a 786-page volume of a yel-
lowed, old, originally multipart philosophy compendium at
a flea market. I began to fill its unread pages with pasted pictures of faces, bodies, buildings, furniture, and clothing I had
collected from *Vogue*, *Harper's Bazaar*, *Elle*, *Cosmopolitan*, and
Architectural Digest. I searched for myself in these magazines

and transferred what I found into my compendium. At Hamburg's main public library, I copied pictures from books; at home I put them in the one book that belonged to me.

In my daydreams I lived inside this anthology, perpetually pasted over with new layers. I closed my eyes and saw myself spending all afternoon at my house, just me and my long, smooth legs. Sometimes I fell asleep imagining my prospects, a smile on my face, my head buried deep in the couch cushions, while my mother did the laundry, chopped, or sautéed. I didn't see her; all I saw was me and my long, smooth legs while my name echoed hollowly from her weary mouth. A name I didn't even recognize in my dream body in my dream house. In my mind, the second I closed my eyes, I became this other woman, whom my mother didn't know.

Whenever I drew the lines of this woman's waist and the blank of her absent nose, I became her. The drawings were secret blueprints, accompanied by a prayer:

> *When I grow up. When I grow up. When I grow up.*
> *When I grow up.*
> *When I grow up. When I grow up. When I grow up.*
> *When I grow up.*
> *When I grow up. When I grow up. When I grow up.*
> *When I grow up.*
> *When I grow up. When I grow up. When I grow up.*
> *When I grow up.*

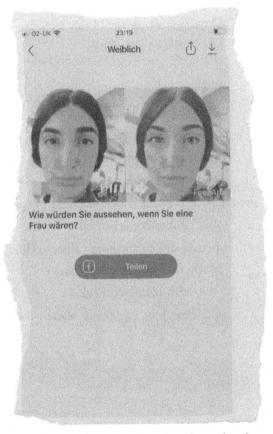

"Feminine" filter in FaceApp face editor designed to show: "What would you look like as a woman?"

DREAM BODY

Daydreams become blueprints,
then battle plans.

A skinny kid doubles over.
She slaps her thighs,
hangs herself up by her hairy armpits.
She scratches her stubbly arms
and puffs up her flat chest.
She takes an axe and chops her nose in two.
One piece is buried,
the other placed in her mother's calloused hands.
Mother, I am going into battle
with blade to cheek,
your daughter under my blade.

IMITATION

How did she hoodwink so many successful people into believing she was something she so clearly was not, the journalist Jessica Pressler asked in a 2018 piece for *New York Magazine*, Anna "Delvey" Sorokin being the "she" in question. Really, though, how did that girl pull it off? In one respect, she reminds me of myself. The flashbacks to the grifter's childhood in the Shonda Rhimes film *Inventing Anna* could portray me, when she is shown sitting on the floor surrounded by glossy magazines, intent on stitching together pictures of other people to create her ideal life. Anna Sorokin was born in Russia in 1991 and grew up as a migrant in Germany. That makes her only two years older than me, so at that age she and I were reading the same magazines, imitating the same It-Girl aura of the early aughts: haughty indifference with jutting shoulders and an angled arm, a purse ideally dangling from the crook, with a pair of enormous sunglasses on the tip of her nose. We intoned the names of designers we couldn't afford. We pored over pictures of the purported lives of the rich and famous and plastered them around in places where we made a ritual of studying them, like the memory of a future that was never promised to us.

In her early twenties, Anna would defraud a host of hotels and banks as well as a friend, who later described her to the media as a sociopath, a narcissist, and a criminal. For a moment she, the white Russian, with her heart-shaped face and pouting lips, gained access to the world of images we as girls both studied on glossy paper. These images asked to be studied and sought after, but we were not to penetrate them. Anna managed to imitate the lives of those she saw, without being one of them. Anna managed to imitate the bearing of a German heiress, which was how she presented, only the actual legacy was missing. Economic capital couldn't be faked. Anna was sentenced to twelve years in prison for fraud in 2019.

Imitation represents a promise of social ascent for some, a survival strategy for others. It can mean we try to disappear in the crowd, mimic normality, dilute ourselves to the point of interchangeability, which frees us from isolation, otherness, and insecurity. The promise of assimilation is the promise of the normalization of our existence. People like Anna, though, so-called grifters, who presume to mimic not normality but exclusivity, do not want to blend in. As a young woman, I couldn't bear the thought either—of not being one of those that our society meant when it told us about the people we should all look up to, fall in love with, watch without envy when they put their fame and fortune on display.

The popular fascination around grift like Anna's arises from the fact that it isn't alien to us. Fraud or deceit as a way of life is required of us daily. We are expected to imitate the collective models presented to us, but evidently every imitation has a threshold. Grift prompts us to ask where the line is: When general self-optimization is based on imitation, when does that veer toward deceit? Where does simple inspiration or fascination with the lives of the haves end and deception begin?

It's no coincidence that imposter syndrome, that gnawing, modern-day feeling of deception, is experienced by so many for whom the wish of social advancement has come true, at least a little, and who now move in spaces and scenes to which their own mother—that embodiment of their social origins—would never have had access. It's the feeling of being fundamentally out of place, as if they didn't deserve to be where they are, to be seen, rewarded, or even loved. It's the feeling that those who have historically been in the majority in all these spaces will see us, that they'll sniff us out and expose us. If they step too close, straightaway they'll see that we're just trying to imitate them, speak their foreign language, wear their clothes as costumes and their smiles as masks—that we aren't one of them. The tale of our mimicry can be subtle and gradual, a slow alienation from the gestures of our own mothers, from the features of our own faces. A discomfort that breaks out like a cold sweat. This terrible fear thrums in the pit of our stomach, knowing that we have to imitate others to get anywhere near the good life.

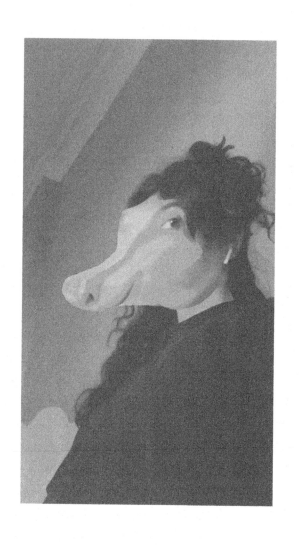

PRETTY MUG

What was hidden behind your pretty mug?
It was always faces like yours
that got away with making faces;
symmetry allowed it.

A smile
stood guard
when our gazes
grazed you lot.

Your prettiness oppressed me.
But oh, how I longed
for the looks and body
that offended me in their plainness,
but promised validation in their echo.

The absence, presence
of gaps and curves,
of the darkness of our brow,
of the thicket on our cheeks—
that alone determined
who garnered forgiving glances
and who went unseen?

I blushed with shame
at my devotion to a beauty
that applied to you
and not me.

What does your pretty mug hide,
in whose contradiction we both reside.

Letting others live and thrive
on one's own rejection—
how embarrassing.

CARTOGRAPHY OF MY UGLINESS

The cartography of my ugliness was a cynical drawing, a depiction I worked on day and night during the era of my pubescent body. I surveyed myself and added lines to the drawing that had not been there a day earlier. I looked in the mirror and erased and drew over the previous lines, which appeared greater and more grotesque with each passing day. I divided my small body into enemy territories. Chemical bleaches were applicable from the hips up, the razor from the hips down.

There was my head, big and unsteady on a twiggy neck and short little body. The face was such a mess, it had barely any room. I gave myself a pointed, cool nose, like a sharp blade, a place where anyone who got too close would cut themselves.

My eyes were glazed and tired, the eyeballs big and intense, the bags under them deep and exhausted. And my mouth became very small and insignificant, parched and alone.

That was the drawing—a cynical reckoning with my body, at once mathematical and militaristic. An honest analysis intended to prepare me for myself. There was no way I would ever be beautiful.

But would I allow myself to be exceptionally ugly? It was one thing to be short, thin, and distinctive, but to be short, thin, distinctive, and hairy—that went beyond excruciating. My battle plan took aim at that last element.

My fur became the scapegoat.

My mustache was striking and, unlike most other parts of my body, could not be concealed. When I spoke, each word was framed by little hairs. And these little hairs deprived me of my femininity. My mustache was thicker and coarser than the fuzz on my chin and cheeks. I could have bleached it to make it less noticeable, but then I would have had to do my whole face. How else could I have explained the transition from blond fuzz to the black hairs that sprouted from every follicle on my brow and the rest of my body?

When my sister was twenty-five, her gynecologist stroked her face and congratulated her: What with your blond hair, if they're lucky, maybe your twins will be blond too. I hadn't been lucky enough to be born blond, nor, for that matter, had my sister, who taught me how to apply a smelly blue cream to my face and fan it with a magazine until my skin stopped burning. The stuff routinely singed patches on my chin and around my mouth. Then, instead of hair, I had small wounds all over. Sometimes I wondered which I preferred: wounds or hair?

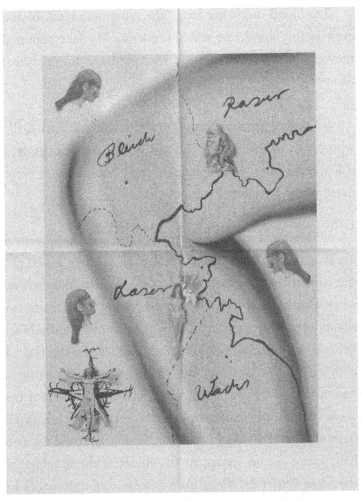

Designations from upper right (thigh): Shave / Bleach / Laser / Wax

The blond didn't last long. The roots were black blazes, even as the blond tips still shimmered. My face appeared unhygienic, dirty. Sometimes I wondered which I preferred: dirt or hair?

If I shaved my mustache, it grew back as stubble, usually within two or three days. But if I shaved too frequently, I risked razor burn. In moments of total desperation, I wondered which I preferred: a rash or hair?

In this way I mapped out my body and declared war on my skin, over and over again. Many of these offensives taught me defensive strategies: a hand at my face to hide behind when I spoke, a twitch in public, a spasm, a hesitation, an abrupt turn away from a companion in the blazing sunshine. Whenever someone looked at me, I felt a stirring fear of chin stubble, impurity, ugliness. I was engaged in a battle as repetitive as it was boring. I would have been furious at the waste of my time and energy, had I not already exhausted both on each individual little hair. When I removed my arm hair, where should I stop? At the elbow, at the shoulder, at the neck? Where did illegitimate hair end and legitimate hair begin? I could have plucked, epilated, or waxed, gone in for laser treatment, professional permanent hair removal. Much as my hair tormented me, though, I couldn't shake the sense that there would be nothing gained in eradicating it.

ALIENATION

All this whiteness that burns me. . . .
I sit down at the fire and I become aware of my uniform. I
had not seen it. It is indeed ugly. I stop there, for who can
tell me what beauty is?

    —**FRANTZ FANON** (trans. Charles Lam Markmann),
      Black Skin, White Masks

In his 1952 study *Black Skin, White Masks*, psychiatrist and anticolonial philosopher Frantz Fanon illuminates the psychological consequences of assimilation in the French colonies. He writes of a white world that presents itself as the only one worthy of respect, that excludes even as it holds the same captive, that demands to be watched, even as it excludes. In his accounting the words *beautiful* and *white* become indistinct, just as the lines blur between *ugly* and *black*. This whiteness, which considers itself beautiful—better, purer, more reasonable, more complete—turns the bodies of others into subordinate "uniforms" in the hierarchy, yet demands that they don white masks. It demands that they imitate. Fanon's profound analyses of colonized patients unearth internalized white norms that manifest in all aspects of the body, even on the surface, the skin. Colonized people learn to view themselves through the contemptuous eyes of the colonizers. Whiteness structures their desires, feelings, bodies, and spirits. Feeling that your own skin is a hindrance, or flawed, becomes an unbearable prison in a uniform that cannot be shed. The relentless representation of the colonized body as that of the criminal, loser, or barbarian burns itself into your retinas. Only to look in the mirror and discover, to your horror, that you are the barbarian. Fanon conceives of ugliness as the trauma of inhabiting a body you have learned to hate: "When it was I who had every reason to hate, to despise, I was rejected?"

Alienated from our bodies, we learn to perceive our lives through the eyes of what the political scientist Benedict Anderson describes as socially constructed "imagined communities." Alienation, a theoretical concept first articulated by Karl Marx, describes the negative effects of private property and capitalist division of labor on the worker. Fanon adopts and elaborates on the term. He demonstrates how the root of colonized people's (self-)alienation is found not only in their economic exploitation but in having their culture redefined for them by external forces.

The victim of cultural imperialism is an alienated person—a person who hates themselves and who imitates their oppressor. In his 1964 essay collection *Toward the African Revolution*, Fanon writes, "The oppressor, through the inclusive and frightening character of his authority, manages to impose on the native new ways of seeing, and in particular a pejorative judgment with respect to his original forms of existence." The oppressor not only rules over the oppressed; he exercises his "inclusive and frightening . . . authority" to manipulate them into hating themselves and their very way of being.

*

Ugliness would be a superficial thing
if it weren't actually about hatred,
about wishing you weren't hated,
didn't hate yourself.

The truth is, we don't want to be more beautiful—
we just want to be fully human.
The closer we think a person comes to beauty,
the closer we figure they come to the full experience
being denied us.

It is for myth that we create ugliness,
this regime and all its uniforms.

It isn't the same hatred, nor the same uniform, that they force on us. This world even has hierarchies for its oppressed, for those excluded and exploited. The symptoms of ugliness divide us every which way, alienated from our own bodies, dazed by the searing whiteness that starts outside our skin and envelops us. The oppressors group us by the hatred of ourselves and others' hatred of us, by our hatred of others, and by the symptoms they give us and that constitute the uniforms of our own individual ugliness.

We learn to see each other, ourselves, and them through a gaze that searches for and seeks distance from ugliness. A construct unfolds, crowned by the very hatred that hates us most. It is this hatred's gaze that stares down our face in the mirror. The gaze that nestles inside us and watches others. It is the hatred occupying and observing us all.

I place the blade to my skin and destroy the evidence.
Even fixing my nose is just a slash of the scalpel away.
Why do I set the blade against my cheek,
when what needs real correction is this hatred?

II. NASAL ANALYSIS

Can one abandon the old nose, with all of its associations? Or, as Nietzsche suggests, is one merely a hypocrite—a person with two noses, one worn in public, one hidden within the psyche?
    —SANDER L. GILMAN, *Making the Body Beautiful:*
    A Cultural History of Aesthetic Surgery

Sixteen-year-old Adolphine Schwarz didn't want to look Jewish. Taking a cue from her older brother, who had already had work done on his nose, she sought out the famed plastic surgeon Jacques Joseph. The rhinoplasty proved far beyond her means, but Joseph generously lowered the price, it being his wish to assist all those afflicted with "Jewish-looking" noses. Schwarz's nose job took place in January 1933, shortly before the National Socialists assumed power, making it one of Joseph's last procedures before Jewish doctors were stripped of their licenses a few months later.

"Joseph the Nose Guy" (*Nasenjoseph*), as the doctor was known, was the son of a rabbi. He was born Jakob Joseph in 1865, died in 1934, and studied medicine in Berlin, where he cast off his Jewish name and became Jacques. During World War I, he took a leading role in facial reconstruction surgeries for disfigured servicemen. When in 1915 the emperor offered him a professorship at the Charité university hospital, on condition that he cast off his faith as well, Joseph declined.

Today Joseph is considered the founder of modern plastic surgery, rhinoplasty in particular. By the turn of the century, he had opened a private practice to offer procedures that his superiors deemed medically unnecessary. He performed his first corrective surgery on a young man who described his nose as a deformity that impaired his social and professional life. Joseph presented the case to the Berlin Medical Society on May 11, 1898, and argued that such medical intervention on a healthy person was "scientifically" justified, as the patient was much happier afterward.

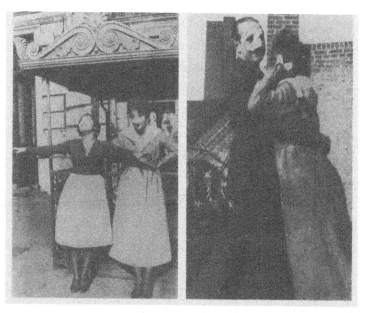

Photos depicting happy patients that appeared in Jacques Joseph's textbook on rhinoplasty.

Later, during the Weimar era (1918–1933), with fewer patients whose faces had been devastated by disease or war, plastic surgeons found they needed new clientele for their services. If one could no longer rely on higher powers or external violence to generate demand, perhaps ideologies or social groupings could help. Joseph's early claim about happiness achieved by means of operative self-optimization would prove instrumental in the rise of aesthetic surgery. It heralded a new philosophy of surgically altering the body that to this day continues to produce ever new forms of manipulation. The notion of physical self-optimization functions as a technical extension of an ideology that upholds the necessity of shaping people into civilized modern citizens. As such, the goal of anatomical correction is not only for patients to become happier in life by attaining a *normal* or *ideal* appearance, but for them to participate more fully in society. The false promise of modern citizenship entails the ability and burden to keep growing, improving, and conforming.

The call for individual self-optimization, hitherto couched in social and political terms, found its way into biology and medicine in the nineteenth century. Alteration as a progressive idea increasingly became the remit of laboratories and operating rooms. Should modern individuals find themselves excluded and unhappy, the onus is on them to change, thus making themselves less deserving of hate. The source of unhappiness is found in the body of the unhappy.

NOSE IN SHADOWS

We trace our big sister's
little nose
with our index fingers.

Until my niece was born
there were four women in our family.
Then there were five, until our mother died.

Four long faces with long noses. I always thought I
looked the least like my mother, because my eyes were big-
ger than hers. As I got older, time and time again I would
draw my fingers across her face. Across a face that gazed at
me, earnest and shy, in the few photos from when she was
young. As I got older, I tried to grow out my hair and part
it in the middle, just as she had in her early twenties. When
she died, I took to wearing her long coats, her soft white
cotton slacks with lace at the ankles, her big rings, her rose
perfume.

My oldest sister told me that two men had made comments about her nose before she eventually decided to have
surgery. She promised herself she would lose her *ugly nose* the
minute she could afford it. One of the men was her supervi-
sor at work. He said:

"You'd be so pretty without that big nose of yours."

The other man was our father. He said:

"What's the matter with you? Your nose gets longer and your face gets narrower by the day. You all take after your mother. You're all your mother's daughters."

I am no stranger to his words. He routinely pointed out what a beak I had sprouted. I was certain my father thought his daughters were ugly. He loved his ugly daughters, but he never failed to remind them how hard it was for him to look past their long faces and long noses.

*

My friend D. told me her husband had remarked in passing that it would be better if their daughter inherited his nose. She was hurt. At the same time, though, her own family had started hoping aloud that the unborn grandchild would get her father's nose. D. couldn't act upset with him; she knew she was loved in spite of, and not because of, her nose. Her mother, her sisters, her aunts, all of them had gotten nose jobs. It was a tradition: you were born with the nose, then you despised it, then you paid for its alteration. D. got the nose and endured the ridicule, but then something happened that alarmed her family: she kept her nose. Sometimes, D.'s mother would fall silent and sigh while they were talking, as though trying to imagine her daughter's face without the nose: "*Aiyyy*, you are so beautiful, but that nose." She would then shake her head theatrically. "*Tsstsstss*, what a waste." Should D. ever reconsider, she would pay for the procedure, mother reminded daughter.

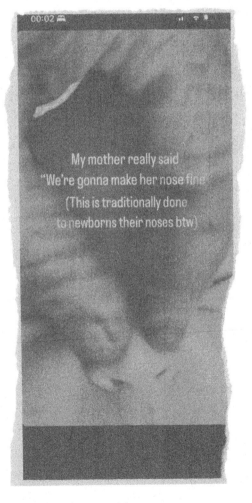

Our big sister underwent plastic surgery when she was twenty-three. She wanted a nose reduction, but her surgeon said he refused to break and reconstruct a *normal nose* for no good reason. A procedure of that nature was too risky, he said, as the nose could shift and end up deformed, so my sister would have to keep coming back for corrective work. A procedure that aggressive could entail a painful, complicated recovery and difficulty breathing for the rest of her life. He would not give her the "Hollywood button nose" she desired, but for five thousand euros he would fix two small details: remove the bump and the drooping tip. The procedure was to be as minimal as possible, meant to repair her *flaws* without looking fake. She later told me:

"People don't question my nose;
they don't question me."

After my oldest sister had her nose done at age twenty-three, at age nineteen my second-oldest sister ran a finger along her own nose. Was she ugly too, another one bound for surgery? I was fifteen years old and studied my profile in the mirror, peering over my shoulder to try to see my face as a stranger might. My second-oldest sister told me she had never thought twice about her nose until our big sister came home bandaged, with swollen dark circles under her eyes:

"I thought
I was ugly and dirty

because I was dark and brown, and you all weren't.
But we all had the nose, until one of us
no longer did."

My second-oldest sister told me people stared in disbelief
when she took our pale little brother to the playground. *That
couldn't possibly be her brother. Is she his babysitter?* This sister
could not help feeling that her skin color was a punishment,
even when our mother stroked her arm and assured her she
wasn't *black*, she was "the color of wheat." It wasn't until she
saw Kajol Devgan spark love and desire in a 1990s Bollywood
romance that the tightness in my sister's chest eased.

*

D. had dressed up as a witch for Carnival one year in grade
school, when a boy came running up to her. He blocked her
way, extended a clammy white hand, and tugged on her plastic nose until her real nose poked out. Then the boy grinned
from ear to ear and whispered:

"You don't even need this."

D. constantly had to be reminded that she had a big
nose. As long as other viewpoints weren't imposed on her,
she never thought about it. When she woke up each morning
and looked in the mirror, she saw a slender nose that was all
hers, exactly where it ought to be. She took a deep breath

and went about her day. When she got pregnant, she gained weight in her face, and everyone watched her features fill out and soften. When her daughter was born, they all held their breath, until the child's face appeared, her nose tiny, and the family breathed a sigh of relief. In the months that followed, D.'s face slimmed down and everyone watched her old features return. She told me:

> "Ever since my daughter was born, I can't stop thinking about my nose. I wonder what other people think when they see us together. Do they breathe a sigh of relief?"

It was in grade school that D. discovered what her nose signified. A Turkish boy came running up to her. He blocked her way, pointed a sticky index finger, and grinned from ear to ear: "You're a Kurd," he said.

"My dad says you can always tell a Kurd by their nose."

From then on, D. attuned her body to the contours of her nose. She vowed never to do it harm. This nose was not to meet the fate of those that came before, those noses belonging to the women in her family. She ran a finger down her nose and whispered:

"I will protect you."

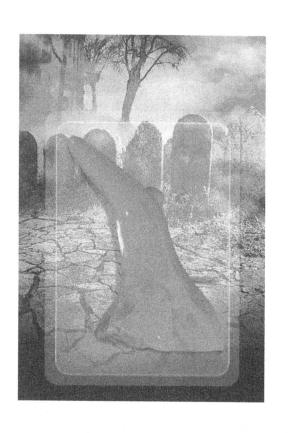

THE LONG-SUFFERING NOSE

The poor nose has long come under fire.

It was targeted as early as the European Renaissance, when any eye-catching nose immediately called syphilis to mind. Given the spread of the sexually transmitted infection, a syphilitic "saddle nose" became a sign of moral depravity and was considered due punishment for the sins committed by those who bore it on their faces. The nose, often left collapsed and ravaged by the disease, became something frightful, whereas it might have been seen as a badge worn by survivors. A person *without a nose* was marked and shunned. True healing meant no scar, no evidence of a surgeon's craft. A scarred nose was a former saddle nose. There must be no reminder that an old nose had ever occupied the same space as the new one.

In the early twentieth century, Jacques Joseph was one of the first in his field to find a surgical solution for minimizing visible scars, which earlier doctors performing skin transplants or other procedures involving external incisions had not managed to achieve. He dominated the discipline, because the visibility of his clients' noses was a serious issue for them. Their noses were inspected, marked, identified, and disparaged as "Jewish noses" or "hooknoses." European society drove them into the arms of the surgeon, who promised relief.

German anti-Semites were obsessed with proving the otherness of Jews. A number of ideologues in the late nineteenth century attempted to gather anthropological evidence for Jews' non-European descent, which could be used to justify their exclusion from the "white race" and thus from Nordic populations. To that end, ethnologists and medical professionals catalogued Jewish skin tone, hair color and structure, and nose shape in an effort to lump Jews together with "races" that were already deemed inferior within the colonial worldview. Of especial interest was always the nose. The German racial theorist Hans F. K. Günther, a major influence on Nazi ideology, went so far as to distinguish between "black" and "white" Jews based on the flat or long noses each supposedly had. Natural scientists studied nasal curvature because they believed a person's origins were revealed in reading their face. Beyond the nose, "Jewish" ears and feet were big pseudoscientific talking points that soon made their way into standard texts on physiognomy and anatomy taught to the German middle class. They constituted the core of a racial theory that relied on outward appearance to determine who was good, bad, healthy, or sick; who was allowed to reproduce and who was not; who was permitted to live and who was not.

*

Only in a world in which the curve of one's nose or flare of one's ears can make a face *different*—a world in which that curve or flare exposes one to the dominant system and its concept of humanity—can surgical intervention be life-altering. Twentieth-century aesthetic surgery promised to change the body in such a way that it appeared *healthy* and thus *racially acceptable*. Early rhinoplasty established the idea that correcting for ugliness wrought by disease, injury, or "race" was medically sound, which paved the way for plastic surgery to spread and develop into the modern discipline that underlies today's beauty industry. Once it became possible to change racialized features that society had believed unchangeable, a whole world of possibilities for physical modification seemed to open. In *Making the Body Beautiful: A Cultural History of Aesthetic Surgery*, the historian Sander L. Gilman writes that the modern promise of assimilation as well as the promise of bodily autonomy were necessarily restricted, because both depended upon a racist model. The more the subject does to change, the more secure the racist model feels in its supposed greater value, its own authenticity as compared to the assimilated subject: "You become a mere copy, passing yourself off as the 'real thing,'" Gilman writes. Accompanying the new nose is the fear of being discovered.

*

Since about 2004, tabloids have run and rerun a pixelated before-and-after image under the headline "Chinese Man Sues Wife for Being Ugly." In this modern-day saga (debunked by the fact-checking website Snopes, though this did little to squelch its viral spread), a man evidently filed a lawsuit against his spouse after she gave birth to an ugly daughter. The judge sided with the plaintiff—"the Court AGREES"—and ordered the woman to pay him $120,000, because she had tricked him into believing she was beautiful.

Reports state that Jian Feng fell in love with his wife for her beauty. A digital photo seemingly battered by countless downloads and uploads shows two blurry female faces with no resemblance. The woman on the right—presumably the person Jian Feng thought he was marrying—has big eyes and a slender nose. She looks artificial, though she supposedly had born a real baby at some point. The woman on the left looks exhausted, or like she didn't put on makeup. There are bags under her narrow eyes. She could be real. We don't need the help of any caption to realize that the left-hand side is before, that *she* is the *Before* in a Before-and-After intended to be read from left to right. As though it went without saying that the Chinese woman with big eyes and a slim nose on the right is the result of a beautifying transformation, as compared to the woman with the small eyes. As though she had broken free of her earlier state, from left-to-right, of course, just like reading Latin script.

When their daughter was born, Jian Feng was reportedly shocked at her appearance, as most of the 624,000 Google results for "Chinese man sues wife for being ugly" claim: "Our daughter was incredibly ugly, to the point where it horrified me," *The Irish Examiner* quoted him as saying. Jian

Feng filed for divorce, accusing his wife of infidelity, only for a DNA test to prove the child was his—the child was theirs, Jian Feng's (whose own features are never described) and his beautiful, beautified wife's, whom he allegedly married out of love and was now trying to divorce on grounds of deceit. The mother's pretty face is revealed as ugly by the birth of her first child. As the German television network RTL put it: "The truth came to light when the girl was born—because no amount of plastic surgery could change his wife's genetic material. His wife was not born with those looks."

*

The term *passing* can describe a person's moving through life unquestioned as someone other than who they truly are. As early as the nineteenth century, the phenomenon was at once a survival mechanism to some and considered a criminal offense to others. When people were accused of passing, it was the act of concealing their "true selves" (which usually meant race) that was so objectionable, because in their hiding the truth, the boundaries of social order were transgressed.

A kind of surgical eugenics emerged in the United States with regard to what was called the "Irish nose." In the 1880s, a surgeon named John Orlando Roe threw himself into developing a new "American nose." Like Jacques Joseph, Roe employed a technique that minimized scarring. He also had at his disposal clients defined by their noses, noses that stood in the way of their assimilation into white mainstream society. When they weren't portrayed as doglike creatures, Irish immigrants in nineteenth-century American caricatures were depicted as something between a Neanderthal and modern Homo sapiens, racist imagery that originated in Great Britain and followed the purportedly backward migrants all the way to the American settler colonies. With the offer of an "American nose," Roe was promising his patients a new nose, yes, but also a degree of invisibility that would liberate them from European tradition.

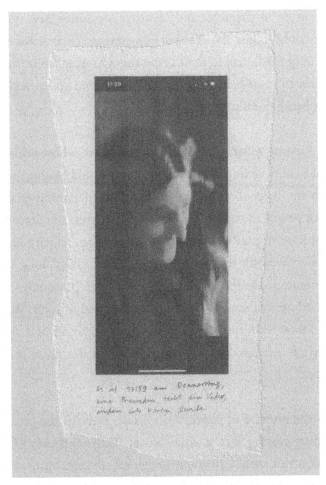

It's 5:59 p.m. on Thursday, a friend shares a video in which I walk by.

In the United States, surgeons like Roe promised Jewish and Irish migrants that they could be physically Americanized, and that corporal change would be accompanied by a transformation in character and identity. A positive new way of life would follow the external adjustment. Their noses were the only roadblock to their being thought of as *white*, that is to say, to their belonging to the hegemonic group without ever being questioned about it.

Anyone whose skin was light colored or whose ethnicity could not be defined beyond any doubt would be able to pass with the help of rhinoplasty. This kind of passing enabled Black people in the United States to transgress the draconian legal lines of political and social segregation, which Gilman cites as a reason the correction of "Black noses" long went unmentioned in the medical literature. Such procedures were carried out, of course, but not documented as such. We do not know who, but we do know that every now and again, someone managed to pass, blending into the norm at first glance.

The promise of plastic assimilation presents the prospect of disappearing into a visual norm. Patients dream of liberation not merely from an imagined conspicuousness, but from having actually experienced stigma for a nose that's too big or too small. The hegemonic class could read an over- or undersized nose as justification for prejudice.

Deviating as they did from the accepted appearance of the white hegemonic class, such noses were loaded and burdensome. Patients begged to become the type of person who could forget about their body. They wanted to become one with those whom they could only imitate. Plastic assimilation was their capitulation.

In biology, the term *assimilation* describes the process of an element being absorbed by a larger organism. Plastic assimilation tricks itself and patients into believing that the modern nation-state is absorbing a given minority—which is doing its utmost to adapt—into the (ethnic) body politic. Unsuccessful assimilation, despite one's efforts, results in feelings of humiliation and shame. We observe the outsider's continual sense of obligation, while the promise of assimilation remains beyond reach. It's more than mere vexation expressing itself in the shame one feels at not being accepted by society, even after giving up one's nose, heritage, and community. The structurally Other cannot employ external simulation to escape entrenched fascist ideology in society. And entrenched fascist ideology is never simply looking to reject the deviant nose as such; it is out to reject the very existence of the human to whom the nose belongs.

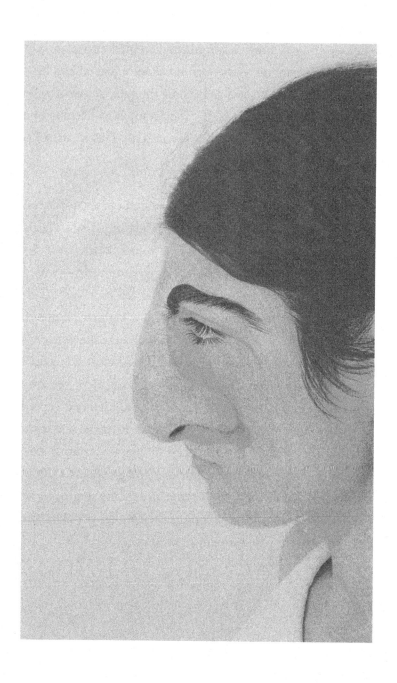

READING FACES

Before I set foot in a room, in walks my nose.

It casts a shadow that engulfs me.
Cloaked in black, I peer from its depths.

Who can see me behind this pillar,
a hiding place for my tenderness.

No one would ever guess at my shy, gentle smile
in the shadow of the colossus hindering me.

A glance over the shoulder, a thrust by my lance of a nose,
prevents my friendly eyes from introducing themselves.

A kiss lost in the shadow of the nose.
A skull, bowed in its arc,
two ends meeting.
An elbow indistinguishable
from a chin, from a nose.

An angle that casts a shadow.
A person, half nose.

I take my face in my hands, wander down my jawbone, graze my teeth with the tips of my fingers, then move them up along my nose. I splay index and middle fingers, as if flashing a peace sign, perfect for poking my eyes. I ram them in hard, hard enough to feel my eyeballs under the lids and imagine gouging them out. My fingers keep moving, tracing my thick eyebrows all the way to my tiny forehead, which couldn't even fit my nose. My fingers range across my skull until they reach the crook of my neck. I know this head. I could probe every last change to it blindfolded. And yet, when my mood is tender, I can't see it at all; my head shrinks before my mind's eye as I soften and grow more delicate. Cramped shoulders, tight jaw—they release. My body becomes at once gossamer and unswerving. My face glows. I can feel myself without wanting to touch my bones. I feel a face that does not belong to me but that lives in my thoughts. It's the face of a nice person, and not mine. I've seen her on TV. She looks straight through the screen, and for a second I think it's a mirror. A second face occupies her face in the reflection; it's the face she's watching, the one watching her. It's my face, spilling over the edges, as though I had engulfed the woman, cast her from the screen. The head that engulfed her is not delicate, and it certainly isn't gentle. My head grows heavy and collapses between my shoulders. My image is heavy and hard, bones protruding at all angles, my chin like a cliffside, teeth set like iron bars, nose like a phallus. I wear a mask. I touch it with my fingers. It belongs to me. My face is a mask.

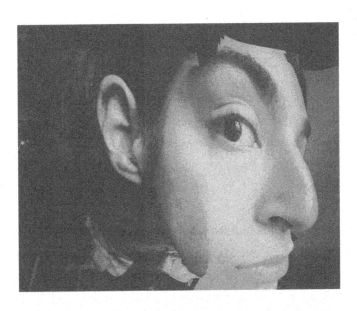

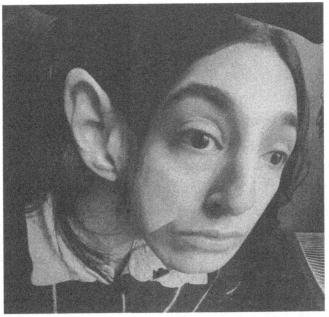

A generic mental image may be considered to be nothing more than a generic portrait stamped on the brain by the successive impressions made by its component images.

—FRANCIS GALTON, "Generic Images," 1879

Charles Darwin's half cousin, Francis Galton, is recognized as the father of eugenics. Galton was interested in the supposed hereditary qualities of intelligence and talent, and in 1883 launched a eugenics movement aimed at targeted human breeding. He developed a range of statistical methods to that end, one of which was combining portraits to serve as visual representations of different human types. Since 1878, Galton had employed multiple exposure techniques on glass-mounted photographic negatives to produce images of superimposed faces. His objective was to display the "average features" of the groups in question, and he would use up to five hundred negatives to create one of his "composite portraits." Those areas that component portraits had in common appeared darkest on the plate, because of their repeated exposure, and suggested "an imagined, hypothetical person," as the art historian Kris Belden-Adams puts it. In her 2020 study *Eugenics, "Aristogenics," Photography: Picturing Privilege*, Belden-Adams writes that this process enabled Galton to endow the "generic mental images" we have of groups of people with an enduring visual form. She describes how diffuse stereotypes that play out as (repeat) impressions in our minds gained what was believed to be an empirical framework and concrete form through Galton's work. He first used prisoner portraits to test whether their facial features could be linked to specific types of criminality. He later broadened his scope, applying the method to other groups that society deemed inferior, including tuberculosis patients, people with mental illnesses, and racialized groups, as in 1883, when he presented his composition of the "Jewish type." To cap off his comparisons, Galton ultimately worked with what he called the "healthy and talented classes," namely white clergymen, scientists, and scholars. His photographs provided tangible visual aids for European discourse on "good" and "bad" breeding.

*

In *Seeing the Insane: A Visual and Cultural History of Our Attitudes Toward the Mentally Ill*, Sander L. Gilman writes that the nineteenth-century discovery of asymmetrical faces in the West first appeared in studies of the institutionalized: researchers determined (or thought they did) that asylum patients all had asymmetrical faces and applied this observation as evidence of insanity. It is remarkable, Gilman notes, that the researchers failed to notice how lopsided their own faces were. Scientists would not conclude that asymmetry is standard in human faces until the twentieth century. The Western moral tradition was characterized by a tendency to

perceive similarities as the foundation for successful relationships. The more similar its members, the more solid a community, which explains why the search for evil was conducted
on the margins or in the Other. Evil was sought in the bodies
of those already condemned, malevolence traced in the faces
of those already confined.

*

Physiognomy is the practice of judging human character
based on physical appearance, especially that of the face. The
term derives from the Greek *physis*, meaning "nature," and
gnomon, for "judge" or "interpreter." When I started drawing portraits, my stated intention was to create faces that,
because of their *distinctive physiognomy*, were not associated
with beauty or other pleasant features.

The faces I had in mind resembled those of the evil step-
mother, strict headmistress, frigid secretary, wicked witch,
or sneaky and stingy neighbor. They also resembled me. I
had never met anyone who both occupied these roles and
looked like me, yet I felt I knew these characters better than
I knew myself. I wasn't cunning or cruel, but when I smiled
in the mirror, I saw them there, all those mean women. They
crawled from the narrow corners of my mouth, which strug-
gled skyward like two hooks, as though I were concealing
something, just like those women. I was reminded of them
whenever my nose and ears rose with my smile, two horns

and a beak sprouting from my face, like a crow perched on the shoulder of a European witch, like a diabolical omen. They were there with me to remind me of my role.

*

The theory of human physiognomy may extend back to Aristotle and ancient Greece, but it was the Reverend Johann Caspar Lavater who revived and modernized the practice in the eighteenth century. Among contemporaries, the Swiss clergyman's *Essays on Physiognomy, Calculated to Extend the Knowledge and the Love of Mankind* was seen as rendering a hitherto speculative realm in the language of empirical, enlightened science. Those who subscribed to his publications included members of the German aristocracy and distinguished figures in civil society, who formed reading groups and met to "Lavaterize," or characterize individuals based on their portraits or silhouettes of their heads. Lavater secured his theory's commercial success by inviting subscribers to submit their own portraits or silhouettes for him to annotate in print. Though physiognomy is today considered pseudoscience, it was extremely popular for a long time.

In his 2004 book *About Face: German Physiognomic Thought from Lavater to Auschwitz*, Richard T. Gray writes about the face as an assumed hermeneutic surface, the history of this ideology, and its impact on modernity. Lavater was convinced that physiognomy would develop into a scientific discipline that could be expressed in mathematical terms. Faces would become data, numbers that could be calculated and evaluated. From there, it wasn't too far to measuring skulls. Hans F. K. Günther, for instance, the Nazi "Race Pope" (*Rassenpapst*) mentioned earlier, adapted the physiognomic gaze into a racist taxonomy that analyzed everything from hair and skin color to nose shape, chin development, eye placement, and even the size and shape of fingers, all of which enabled National Socialist racial ideology to emerge.

It's disturbing to recognize strains in Günther's argumentation that one hears today with regard to ugliness. For instance, *Rassengünther* ("Günther the Race Guy"), as he was also known, stated that Germans had a natural instinct in their blood that explained their negative response toward black-haired people with pointy noses. I constantly encounter the notion that our reaction to the outward form of the Other is instinctual. It's in everyday life, in political debate, in myself, everywhere.

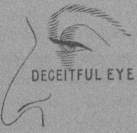

DECEITFUL EYE

An eye like this will represent a character that is positively deceitful. Why not use your own eyes and not be deceived by such?

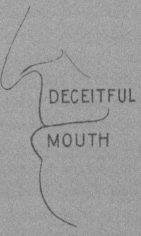

DECEITFUL MOUTH

One with a mouth like this can be very agreeable and still have the most selfish ax to grind.

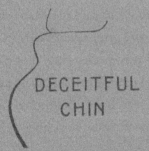

DECEITFUL CHIN

Study this chin young ladies and gentlemen and do not depend too much upon the constancy of anyone with a similar chin.

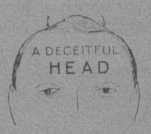

A DECEITFUL HEAD

Clearly remember this shape and apply it.

We lived in Hamburg. Every morning I took the bus to Hagenbeck Zoo, where I had to transfer to the subway to get to school. Every morning I looked at the dark-green bars separating me from the animals' prison that in the nineteenth century was even used to exhibit humans from distant European colonies. As we sped past, the bars blended in with the green of the bushes. Every morning my eyes wandered along the fence, until the bus turned at the entrance to the zoo; until our paths forked. There was a girl I saw on the bus every morning. Sometimes she sat across from me, sometimes just two or three rows away. From the corners of my eyes, I studied her thick eyebrows, which met in the middle and rained down at the edges, delicate as the stroke of a wing and the tips of two feathers. Morning after morning, I reveled in peering at her big, pointy nose, which she flashed in the crowd. Did the girl see me too? On days she wasn't on the bus, I pictured her earnest eyes and grim gaze. If only I could give her a nod one day, like bus drivers did when they passed by in opposite lanes, or like two melanin-rich residents of an otherwise pale city, who could readily put themselves in the other's shoes. I would look her in the eyes, nod, and, without opening my mouth, say:

"I know."

And she would accept the gesture and return it. Maybe I would take her by the shoulders when we got off the bus at the zoo, whisper:

"You are beautiful,"

then dissolve into the crowd. I would never place my hands on her cheeks, such that her face rested in my palms. I wouldn't slowly bring the tip of my nose to touch hers either. I would not close my eyes and imagine an elegant arch forming between two noses that, though they had never spoken, knew each other. I wouldn't do any of that.

Every morning I saw her, I saw myself too, until I never saw her again. One morning I got on the bus and found an empty seat, when in the distance I noticed an unusually familiar-looking girl. She looked like my girl, but then again she didn't. The middle of her face, the spot where everything came together, was alien to me. I felt suddenly uneasy and overheated. Who had done that to her, who had stolen her nose? A terrible loneliness spread down my arms and legs. I couldn't take my eyes off her, until I lost her in the crowd and never saw her again.

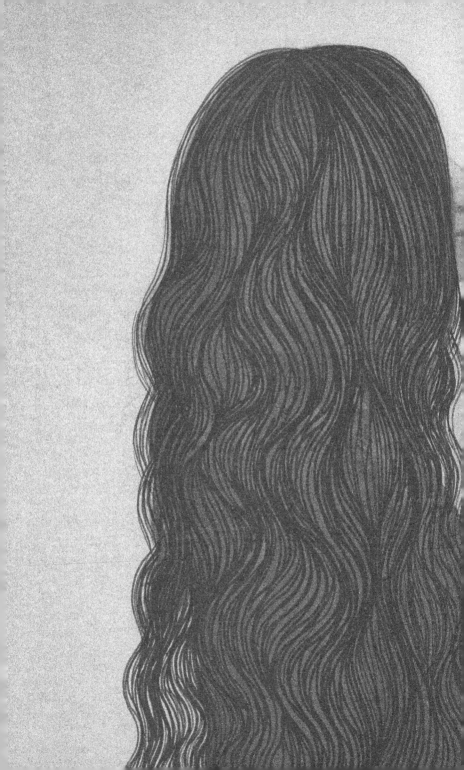

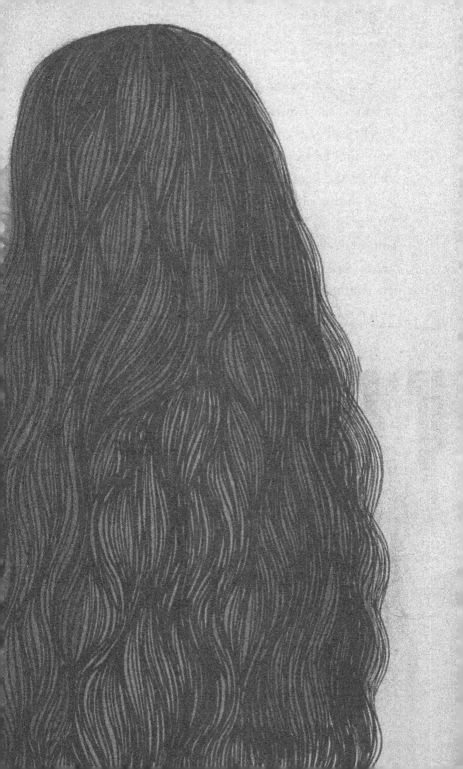

In the early 1870s, the Italian physician Cesare Lombroso examined the remains of a man named Giuseppe Villella. Villella had been imprisoned for theft and arson for many years until his death, whereupon his body fell into the doctor's hands. Lombroso noticed an indentation in Villella's skull. In this indentation, he believed he had uncovered the "nature of the criminal." He compared Villella's skull, jaw, and cheekbones to those belonging to "savages" and "inferior beasts." According to Lombroso, several shared features made the criminal a "perverse, malicious, bloodthirsty" creature; such was his alleged discovery.

European histories of knowledge have many fathers. One such father was Lombroso. His pseudo-anthropological approach to criminology helped establish delinquency as a focus of medical and biological research in the late nineteenth century. Lombroso's work merged supposed discoveries in the field of physiognomy with the misanthropic theories of social Darwinism and the phrenologist Franz Joseph Gall's racist study of skulls. The Nazis would later use his findings to advocate the forced sterilization of "criminals" and the "mentally ill." In the United States, Lombroso provided inspiration to lawmakers in the 1920s as they drafted immigration legislation to grant selective access.

His ideas were in part responsible for altering the modern Western image of evil. Whereas humans had been granted free will and personal responsibility for their actions (in theory, at least) since the Enlightenment, Lombroso argued that villainy was innate and inscribed in the face. The search for the root of evil in the body continues today, even if the focus has shifted from noses and skulls to brains and thought patterns, as when neurological and psychological studies are conducted to determine whether psychopathic tendencies can be detected at an early age. Born criminals were beyond saving, Lombroso believed, and the only reasonable way to deal with them was to remove them from society. He outlined facial features meant to correspond to specific types of crime: Thieves had distinctive faces with bushy eyebrows, crooked or flattened noses, and thin beards. Rapists had delicate features, though their lips and eyelids were swollen, their ears stuck out, and they occasionally had a hunchback. It's no wonder these descriptions sound familiar. We still see them today in depictions, caricatures, and costumes of bad guys in books and film and elsewhere, all of which contribute to our notions of embodied evil. We know the criminals Lombroso invented before we ever come into contact with criminality.

*

Cesare Lombroso's Museum of Criminal Anthropology originated in the nineteenth century, but its Turin premises were shuttered for decades until 2009, when the University of Turin reopened it. A year passed before protesters started calling for the museum to return the human skulls on display to their descendants for proper burial. Many of the nearly seven hundred skulls in the collection were those of poor laborers from southern Italy. They were labeled *Thief, Murderer, Fraud, Bandit,* or *Prostitute,* and Lombroso considered *Rebellion* and *Treason* criminal categories as well. He had developed his concepts during the creation of the Italian nation-state and brutal suppression of political resistance in southern Italy. This father of criminology thus provided a foundation for the racist "criminal" profiling and police record-keeping practices that targeted not only southern Italians, but racialized people generally.

"The development of machines that are capable of performing cognitive tasks, such as identifying the criminality of a person from their facial image, will enable a significant advantage for law enforcement agencies and other intelligence agencies to prevent crime from occurring in their designated areas."

> **-JONATHAN W. KORN**, New York Police Department veteran, Harrisburg University Ph.D. student, and contributing researcher (with professors Nathaniel J. S. Ashby and Roozbeh Sadeghian) of "A Deep Neural Network Model to Predict Criminality Using Image Processing"

In June of 2020, more than one hundred fifty years after Lombroso's examination of the late arsonist and thief Giuseppe Villella, an open letter to the international scientific publisher Springer Nature was published online. Scholars from across disciplines drafted the letter, titled "Abolish the #TechToPrisonPipeline." In it, they decried a forthcoming Springer publication that they argued represented a greater body of computer-aided research and how such findings are being treated. Researchers within this burgeoning field claim to be able to predict "criminality" based on biometric and/or criminal legal data, the letter states. For one, the authors wrote, such claims are scientifically unsound, and secondly, they are part of a political agenda to implement machine learning and artificial intelligence "as a means of depoliticizing state violence and reasserting the legitimacy of the carceral state."

Black scholars have headed the resistance to law enforcement agencies' embrace of new technologies. Although Springer Nature canceled the book deal, concerns persist for the Coalition for Critical Technology (CCT), which penned the letter. The group offers us a reminder that new technologies are reviving old assumptions that science should have scuttled for good a long time ago.

It is impossible, CCT contends, to capture the criminality of a person in a biometric photo or facial scan. In underlying assumptions about society, "criminality" is a notoriously racist category, as is any analysis purporting to predict it.

The desire for science-based criminal recognition is fundamentally corrupt—it robs humans of free will. We all make decisions both in spite of and because of our circumstances, and contained within that tiny *in spite* is our freedom, which cannot be quantified. There isn't a statistical probability calculation or database that can ever rob us of our capacity to defy expectations. And yet, criminalized contexts are not those that technology seeks to detect in the distance between our eyes, but those that surround us. The reality outside our bodies is what creates criminality, not our bodies themselves.

*

Here's a realistic dystopia to contemplate: Kids have their school pictures taken, and a program generates an educational plan for them based on their facial contours. Our faces are read like digital code, the shape of our forehead or nose becoming the qualitative data used to categorize us. This dystopia surpasses any stereotyping or laziness in the habitual way we look at each other that contributes to mutual judging; it describes a fear of a systematic institutionalized prejudgment that's packaged as *progressive* because it employs the vernacular of science and digital technologies, which are supposedly objective. If the plastic surgeons of the nineteenth and twentieth centuries were "helping" people assimilate to a white conception of humanity, what will doctors in this dystopia choose as their models and self-proclaimed goals? In their field, a perfect face would be one that does not provide cause for systematic hatred. A face that would simply be read and rake in positive reviews. In a world where perfect, noncriminal faces are available for purchase, diagnostic facial recognition becomes a tool for regulating the poor, who can't afford the price tag. Physiognomy becomes a further means of cementing economic difference, of dividing up the classroom, of dividing into classes.

PLASTIC

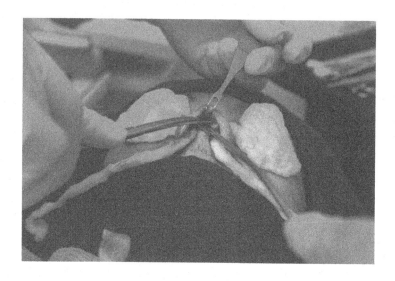

The beautiful dream that we might be freed of pain has become reality. Pain, that greatest perception of our earthly existence, that clearest sign of the imperfection of our bodies, must now submit to the power of the human mind, to the power of ether vapor.... Through [its power], our path to death is half traveled, death itself only half as horrible.

—JOHANN FRIEDRICH DIEFFENBACH,
Der Aether gegen den Schmerz (Ether Against Pain)

The differentiation between unnecessary and necessary medical interventions is key to differentiating between cosmetic surgery and reconstructive plastic surgery. Gilman places the origins of the debate sometime in the late sixteenth century, when syphilis was spreading across Europe and doctors began repairing faces disfigured by the infection. *Chirurgia decoratoria* was initially concerned with the restoration of diseased noses. In 1798 Pierre Joseph Desault coined the term *plastic surgery*, based on the Greek *plastikos*, for "malleable." Twenty years later, Carl Ferdinand von Graefe published a monograph titled *Rhinoplastik*, which set the course for a notion that would lodge itself in my adolescent brain many years later—self-improvement starts with the nose.

In *Allure* magazine's "The Complete Guide to Rhinoplasty" from 2018, board-certified plastic surgeon Adam Kolker outlines what the ideal candidate for a nose job might look like:

You were born with a bump at the bridge of your nose. Your nasal width does not fall within the norm, i.e., your nose is too wide or too narrow. Your nose is asymmetrical, "twisted or deviated," which could disrupt the balance and structure of your face. You have a prominent nasal tip that is "round, bulbous, fatty, or disproportionate to the rest of your face." Or the tip of your nose droops, which Kolker describes as when the angle between your upper lip and nasal tip is less than ninety degrees. According to the experts quoted in the piece, these various criteria add up to eligibility for cosmetic intervention. In other words, they are all *measurable* criteria that can be employed to assess the ugliness of a nose and recommend procedures that are utterly superfluous, medically speaking. Another plastic surgeon calls the initial consultation for prospective clients "the most honest 30 minutes of their life." No one will ever be as honest as a cosmetic surgeon, who can attest to the scope of your ugliness. During that same consultation, the doctor will make you an offer: here's what modern medicine and technology can do to correct the identified flaws, and here's how much it will cost. The expert morphs your photo on an iPad. He models your face, your nose, like clay.

*

Even in the earliest days of rhinoplasty, Jacques Joseph conceived of the plastic surgeon as a sculptor and looked to the art world for direction. One of his role models was the Prussian classical illustrator and sculptor Johann Gottfried Schadow. In his 1835 publication *National-Physiognomien oder Beobachtungen über den Unterschied der Gesichtszüge und der äußeren Gestalt des Körpers* (National Physiognomies or Observations of the Difference in Facial Features and the Outward Build of the Body), Schadow presented various drawings and studies, including some that divided the face into six units, with the admonition that the nose should occupy no more than three. I have tried to recall whether it was Schadow's segmentation of the face that we studied in high school art class and had to use on our self-portraits. In any case, I remember those three segments intended to contain my nose, and how tight they felt when its tip spilled over the line. My forehead, meanwhile, was smaller than it should have been, disproportionate to my nose. I erased the lines that represented my face and corrected them, fitting them into the grid on the sheet in front of me. It looked like someone had squashed my face; perhaps the person in the portrait was an estranged distant relative? I took the drawing home and showed it to my big sister. She rolled her eyes without pausing her search for the remote control. "The same thing happened to me," she said, unmoved. "I painted a self-portrait in my honors art class, and the teacher told me to fix the chin, because it was too long." When my sister held up her reference photo to the painting to compare, her teacher flinched in embarrassment: "Oh, well, if that's your chin, then you can hand in the painting as is."

*

The German Bundestag's art outreach program cosponsored an exhibit in 2016 of "portraits of people from Syria, Afghanistan, or North Africa," held at Schadow Haus, the sculptor's former residence and now a state administrative building in central Berlin. The show featured images of people housed in German refugee centers, waiting for their right to asylum. According to the program, the exhibit was inspired by Schadow's interest in the "tremendous variety of human facial features" and in creating portraits of "foreigners," like the drawing he did of the first Native Hawaiian to visit Prussia. Another aim of the exhibit—and fully in line with Schadow's philosophy—was to demonstrate how much one could learn about "foreigners" by looking at their pictures: "Portraits provide clues about the personality and life of the subject; they can tell us about a person's profession, heritage, and social station." The Bundestag called its display of images of asylum seekers *vis-à-vis: Gesicht zeigen!* ("vis-à-vis: Show Your Face!")

> Show your face!
> No papers, but *illegal* stamped
> across your eyebrows, metrically spaced.
> Hands up, foreigner!
> We're here; you're there.
> Hands up and show your face, foreigner;
> your nose is a dead giveaway—
> not from here.

*

Dr. Rady Rahban of Beverly Hills pops up on my phone: a plastic surgeon with slicked-back hair and a patrician face, without a doubt his family's pride and joy. He wears a black turtleneck sweater under a checkered blazer and has a large, elegant nose that makes him look smarter and wealthier. It's also pretty cheeky, given he makes a living performing nose jobs. Rahban thinks of himself as an artist and sculptor. He builds noses that won't collapse a year later; their structure will hold up for decades. He builds natural, customized noses that match the face, gender, and, most importantly, the ethnicity of his patients. In fact, the term for such procedures is "ethnic rhinoplasty." The name indicates that noses reveal more about a person than they might like. It also shows what's behind the alteration: a distancing from one's heritage, an attempt to escape genetic inheritance, be it broad nostrils or a hooked nose.

Rahban describes it in more dignified, if contradictory terms, right under the "Ethnic Rhinoplasty" header: "Whatever your ethnicity," if you are seeking this corrective work, "it is because you are unhappy with the size, shape and/or function of your nose." According to Rahban, ethnic rhinoplasty is one of the most individualized cosmetic procedures. He promises his patients—his clients—that their "cosmetic goals and needs" will be addressed without erasing their "ethnic identity," an identity found in the nuanced contours and curves of the nose. Rahban says his is "exacting, artistic work." I imagine him being nicer toward noses than other surgeons, with a greater appreciation of their many forms, an appreciation reflected in his own extraordinary nose. I can't decide whether his big nose secures my trust or serves as an admonition against the assimilation that every last one of his procedures signifies. Why is he so confident about his nose, and would I be compelled to have him doctor mine if I lived in Beverly Hills? He answers my tacit question in one of his marketing videos: "a man's nose is different than a woman's nose."

*

The ethnic rhinoplasty Rahban and his cohort are practicing these days traces back to a movement in cosmetic surgery that began in the 1970s. Surgeons back then wanted to shake off the racist history of their discipline, which entailed imitation of white ideals and largely worked on racialized patients to remove ethnic features from their faces. The new movement defined beauty within the respective aesthetic parameters of different ethnicities and developed specific ideals for each. The aim was no longer to sell a nose like a Roman sculpture or out of a German anatomy lesson to an ethnically ambiguous person; it was to provide socially acceptable noses that were proportionate to a person's face. How one defines *proportionate* or *acceptable*, however, remains true to the ideals and norms found in the old textbooks: wide noses should be narrower, big noses smaller, flat noses lifted.

*

Men like Rahban are always popping up in my feed. They reveal work that celebrities have had done to their bodies and faces and tell us that nothing is natural anymore, that everything is a product or service that they happen to offer as well. Rahban has made a name for himself online as a plastic surgeon whose patients' well-being matters more to him than his bottom line. He has an "uncensored" podcast that he hopes will educate people, so they can make informed decisions about their bodies. Plastic surgery, he says, is no longer exclusive to the rich and famous; it's affordable now, more widespread and less stigmatized than in the past. One could even say that the practice is gradually becoming normalized. On another podcast, Rahban chats with the host, who posted a video of their conversation on YouTube and TikTok, because her face deserved to be seen, as she says in the intro. During their talk, he serves up the "brutal truth about plastic surgery." He describes clients who say they don't mind their appearance; they just don't like the way they look in photos. He tells them their noses look fine—then they point to a picture of themselves they hate. He tries to ground them in reality, but they keep going back to the photo. The podcast host holds a hand to her open mouth, trying to look aghast and hot at the same time. But that's crazy, she protests, totally unimaginable.

> "We don't live in the photo,"
> Rahban reminds his patients.
> "That's an angle."
> —An angle that casts a shadow.

Rahban reminds his patients that they are multidimensional creatures in motion, not flat photos, not static objects that can only be viewed from one angle. He seems concerned about the fact that more and more patients want to look exactly like photos on their smartphones. Photos altered by camera filters and editing features, which they have gotten used to over time. Pictures that acquaint them with a face on a screen that cannot be recreated in the mirror without his help:

> We rework our images
> until they no longer match our faces,
> until they become the faces of others,
> until we fit our faces into their pictures,
> until our faces fit the frame.

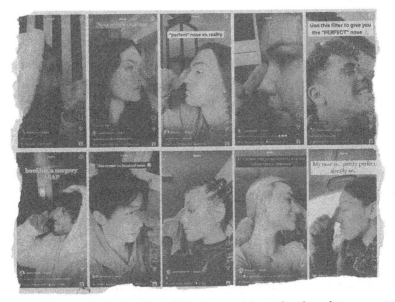

The "Nose Profile Challenge" on TikTok has users place a thumb on their nose, and in 3 ... 2 ... 1 ... lift the thumb to reveal whether their nose is "perfect" or not, whether there's a bump hidden there, or the nose follows the line of the thumb in a graceful curve.

The eighteenth-century Dutch physician Petrus Camper developed a theory of the "facial angle" ascertained by drawing a horizontal line from the nostril to the ear and a perpendicular line from the upper jaw to the forehead. Employing this technique, used then as now to measure the condition of a bulging jaw known as prognathism, Camper concluded that the facial angle of an orangutan was less than sixty degrees; the facial angle of people from Asia or Africa was around seventy, that of Europeans was about eighty, and that of Greco-Roman statues was between ninety and one hundred. Lines like these start at our facial features and carve into our dignity. Lines like these are still felt as we place a thumb on our nose in front of our phone camera. Camper did not propose purely aesthetic standards for the proportionality of our faces. Instead, what he defined with the lines he drew down our noses was the divide between humans and animals. Consequently, every last measurement was marked by another line, at the start of which Europeans placed themselves. The lines of dehumanization run along our edges, on our skin, through our flesh.

*

The Jewish surgeon Jacques Joseph used his non-Jewish wife to illustrate the ideal female face. He justified this choice by highlighting the resemblance between her profile and nose and a drawing by Leonardo da Vinci, in direct reference to the Greco-Roman profile in art, with its thirty degree angle between the nasal tip and chin. Joseph also drew from Albrecht Dürer, the venerated Renaissance painter who so exemplified "German high culture." In the latter half of the nineteenth century, Dürer was co-opted by German nationalists—and soon by National Socialists—who celebrated him for creating the Germanic type and laying the visual groundwork for Germany's national self-discovery. Furthermore, Joseph worked with models developed by the anatomist and physiologist Ernst Brücke, who taught at the University of Vienna and Berlin's Academy of Fine Arts. Brücke published a handbook in 1891 titled *Schönheit und Fehler der menschlichen Gestalt* (*The Human Figure: Its Beauties and Defects*). In it, he details a normative image of the body also based on classical aesthetics. According to Brücke, a woman's body is perfect when pubescent, unmarred by childbirth but fertile and ready for pregnancy. The perfect male body is uncircumcised, the bridge of a man's nose "straight and flush with the forehead, not set at an angle to it, nor separated from it by a depression." Brücke's descriptions of the human form span seven chapters covering head and neck, belly, back, pelvis, elbows, and feet. He also elaborates on human figures he deems "useless" to sculptors.

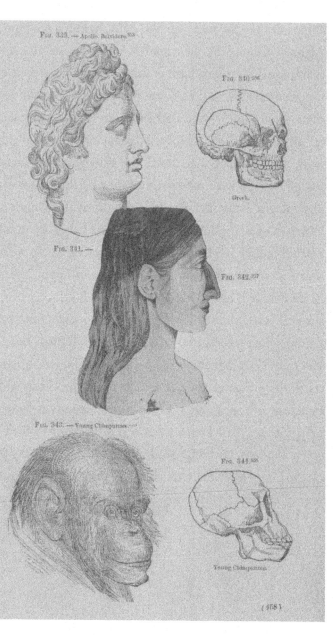

FIG. 340. — Apollo Belvidere.

FIG. 340.

Greek.

FIG. 341. —

FIG. 342.

FIG. 343. — Young Chimpanzee.

FIG. 344.

Young Chimpanzee.

(458)

When Brücke discusses the human form in terms of Greco-Roman ideals, he doesn't mean the actual features of ancient Greek or Roman people—he is referring to the creations of classical artists. The "aquiline nose," for instance, is quite common in Italy, yet it has not been recognized as a form of feminine beauty in art. It was never documented, meaning an Italian woman in Rome might have been born with a hooked nose that was denied representation in idealized Roman sculpture or painting. Brücke's image of beauty embraced the Kantian notion of "classical" perfection and applied it to contemporary society. Joseph adopted this premise for his surgical practice. The bodies he shaped were modeled after figures regarded as irreproachable according to the racial aesthetics of the period.

Idealizing mimicry as an artistic virtue helps invalidate notions of authenticity and the immutability of human nature. Although abandoning the idea of an immutable body could allow for autonomy and the freedom to change, this possibility is limited by the premises of imitation—by the demand for aesthetic assimilation.

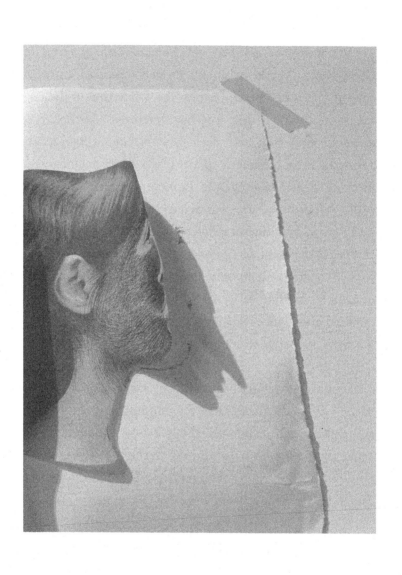

She might have been beautiful, but for her nose.

An actress was supposed to have her nose done. The lights cast an unfortunate shadow on the spot just above her mouth, like a dark little beard reaching from the tip of her nose over her upper lip.

The ideology of proportionality, symmetry, and the supposed harmony of human anatomy limits natural form, just as it intends to optimize it. This ideology was established by men, who by their own metrics would have been ugly, yet who produced templates and models to patent and monitor *superordinate beauty*. It is not overstating the point to describe their attention to idealized Kantian aesthetics, then implemented on the human body, as obsessive.

Why were *ugly* (according to the very rubrics they proposed) men working so doggedly to circumscribe *beauty*? Was their control over the knowledge of beauty an attempt to possess it? As individuals perhaps routinely denied beauty, was the idealization of exclusive features a source of satisfaction? If beauty was out of reach for them, should the same go for everyone else? It would be at once amusing and tragic if the beauty ideals that still haunt us today could be traced back to the asinine resentment of old white men. Nevertheless, their thinking must have been influenced by these, or similar, feelings. In fact, it is imperative that we challenge the avowed objectivity of their writings, that we contextualize that self-declared "objectivity" within these men's biographies. Taken together, however, their words amount to more than just the hateful or insulting musings of individuals in the past.

Taken together, they form an ideological system that could only spread so successfully, and last so long, because there was collective interest in limiting beauty and dehumanizing anyone defined as *not* beautiful. Exclusive beauty represents such a tiny minority that the beautiful can scarcely be considered agents of this stratification. They just happen to benefit from a system maintained by others. The political success of beauty, therefore, does not come down to a small subset of people put on display as role models. Exclusive beauty is effective because it generates the Not Beautiful. Their debasement, their exclusion, and ultimately their dehumanization is the real point of modern concepts of beauty. The production of ugly, sick, or abnormal bodies and the partial or total negation of beauty in the Other enables their exploitation by so-called civilization. The exclusion and exploitation of the many is made possible by the adulation of the few.

Even bodies marked as beautiful do not necessarily profit most from this economy; instead, it's those who set, regulate, and sell these standards, as it always has been. It is those who profit from *the ugly* by preserving the fear of ugliness and disdain for it, so that people will do whatever it takes not to get too close.

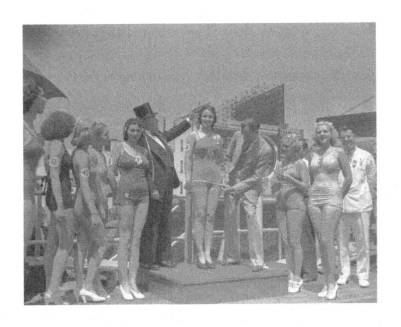

REPRODUCIBILITY

A mother says to her child, "How can I respond to you, when it's my nose on your face, my black hair growing from your skin. You are perfect. I will love you as long as I'm not you." She looks away.

"I cannot escape myself.
My womb bore that which is no longer me."

*

Iran has the highest rate of nose jobs worldwide.

Between eighty and ninety percent of patients are women.

In his 2006 essay "Diffusion of Cultural Models, Body Transformations and Technology in Iran," the sociologist Didier Gazagnadou links this boom in rhinoplasty directly to the images of "Western noses" in circulation there. He sees a connection between today's mass demand for cosmetic surgery and the influence of "women in the entourage of the shah," who in the 1970s imitated certain Western styles as part of general modernization programs in Iran before the Islamic Revolution.

Pierre Bourdieu writes in *Distinction: A Social Critique*

of the Judgement of Taste (1979) that the production of taste is part and parcel of symbolic class warfare. We transmit aesthetic codes that communicate our class background, the French sociologist argues, in how we choose to adorn our bodies and how we (or our faces) present. In this act of negotiation, what we decide to consume is not limited to material goods but permeates our bodily practices, all the way to modifying our bodies and faces. The not wealthy aspire to upward mobility—or at least the semblance of upward mobility, the association with it—in everything from selecting a nice suit for special occasions to investing in a new nose for their daughter.

The anthropologist Sara Lenehan interviewed surgeons and patients for her 2011 study "Nose Aesthetics: Rhinoplasty and Identity in Tehran" and found that many think of big or distinctive, unaltered noses as *aqabmânde* (underdeveloped), *dehâti* (provincial), and *amale* (working class). In the socio-cultural study "'Kill Me but Make Me Beautiful': Harm and Agency in Female Beauty Practices in Contemporary Iran," one of the women surveyed explains that, because of hijab and full-body covers, a nice face is more important than a good body. This means that Westernization alone cannot explain the obsession with rhinoplasty in Iran; at this point, it has become a practice particular to that place. Women in Iran today no longer look to German or Italian faces as models, but instead embrace the ideal of a modern, affluent Iranian, which is how they wish to be perceived.

Although the "European nose" remains a standard surgical model (achieved by reducing overall size, removing the bump, and lifting the tip), it has now been inscribed in the "modern Iranian face." Bleach blond Iranians with button noses do not conflict with the image urban Iranians have of themselves; rather, they represent a homegrown aesthetic. The local economy has helped the spread, and Iran's vast and affordable surgical industry also draws in members of the diaspora for corrective procedures. In speaking with pharmacists in Iran, Lenehan learned that they routinely sell bandages to young men and women who can't afford nose jobs but pretend to have gone under the knife. It would seem that the mere association with rhinoplasty in public is a status symbol if bandages are all it takes to achieve the desired effect.

*

Bella Hadid is the most influential fashion model of my generation. According to a study by the plastic surgeon Julian De Silva, Hadid is the "most beautiful woman in the world," hands down. De Silva found her face to be 94.35 percent accurate to the golden ratio, also known as the *divine proportion*, as implemented by Renaissance painters to achieve *visual perfection*. Like so many men before him, De Silva ran through the battery of requisite measurements, assessing the size and position of eyebrows and eyes, nose, lips, chin, and jaw, among other features. As he sees it, the world's most beautiful woman is the one who most closely matches these measurements: a woman with a wildly above-average symmetrical face.

Hadid is the daughter of a Dutch mother and Palestinian father. In an interview with *Vogue* in 2022, she revealed that she regrets the nose job she had when she was fourteen. She admitted that she had long thought herself ugly, compared to her blond older sister, who is also a model: "I wish I had kept the nose of my ancestors. . . . I think I would have grown into it." There is a lot of speculation online about other procedures she may have undergone. Bella's face is discussed at length by laypeople and plastic surgeons alike: Can a surgically altered face even count as the ideal of human beauty? Shouldn't real beauty be natural?

A good number of plastic surgeons report that they have begun producing Kim Kardashian lookalikes; in an analogy to the language of infectious disease, Kardashian is now referred to as "Patient Zero." Kardashian denies having had several procedures. In response to questions about her nose, she tweeted: " . . . [You] will see when I have kids, they will have the same nose as me." Kardashian's youngest sister, Kylie Jenner, meanwhile, regrets the work she has had done: "I wish I'd never touched anything to begin with," she expressed in a conversation on the reality TV show *The Kardashians*, saying she didn't ever want her daughter to do the things she has done to change her face: "I see my features in my daughter . . . [My] daughter looks like me." Jenner finally sees her own beauty in her child, a perspective missing in the past when she looked in the mirror.

The philosopher Heather Widdows writes about beauty as a dominant ideal and obligation in her 2018 study *Perfect Me: Beauty as an Ethical Ideal*. At the heart of today's globalized beauty ideal is an "imagined self" found as pure potential within the body and the path toward this self. The imagined self is a version we visualize at the end of a transformative beautification and self-optimization process, like the "after" picture in a before-and-after makeover, glow-up, or surgery. We perceive our *actual* bodies as objects—projects—and over-identify with the bodies we want to have. The prospect of a *better*, more beautiful (or even just *good enough*) "me" motivates the subject to endure the consequences and pain that the path to beauty involves, because waiting at the end of that path is the "real self." Widdows writes that the notion of leading a better life as the beautiful, imagined self—however unrealistic or unattainable this may be—is motivation enough for us to follow "beauty regimes."

Identifying with the imagined self splits our consciousness and continually conditions us to engage in critical self-evaluation that juxtaposes our actual bodies, warts and all, with an ideal, imagined body. Widdows argues that we endure the disparity between the real and imagined self because beauty, like an ethical ideal, points us in a specific direction. Though we may never achieve the ideal, we take our cues from it, honoring it through practices and rites that follow set models and give structure to everyday life.

Reading Widdows, I can't help but see my imagined self, which has haunted me my entire life. It's like a torture device, this template I have held up time and again to check how much longer I need to spend in my transitional body before I finally grow into my real body, before I undergo metamorphosis. I remember daydreams in which I would slip into a tubful of bleach or permanent depilatory cream, then emerge with a thinner, softer, smoother body. I can still see my imagined self in these many intimate scenes I couldn't stop picturing, in which I led a desirable, happy, successful life. I call this idealized person "the other woman," a woman with whom I'm cheating on myself, whenever I secretly promise her a better life than the one promised to the self and body I'm actually spending my life with.

Widdows warns that contemporary beauty ideals cast ugliness as personal failure, putting the onus on the individual to strive for beauty. Oftentimes, though, the goal isn't even to reach an ideal, but simply to achieve normality—a labor-intensive and costly normality whose growing demands edge it closer and closer to the unrealistic ideal. The more that broad participation in extreme beauty practices is normalized, the more dominant the ideals they represent become; we see this in the imitation of physical youth, as outward signs of aging in the body are read as failure. The more women seek out Botox, laser treatments, fillers, or chemical peels, the more normalized and thus compulsory these new technologies become for *all* women who want to be seen as put-together, healthy, and not ugly.

If such normalization occurs, wrinkles or even visible pores will attract as much negative and embarrassing attention as body hair already does for so many. For a long time now, public figures who forgo cosmetic interventions and instead "age naturally" have been considered an exception, not the rule. Showing wrinkles will soon be seen as a political decision or statement, just as it has become a feminist, politically coded move since the end of the twentieth century for women to show—and not to shave—their underarm hair. As it becomes easier and more effective to mask signs of aging, will it become even easier to identify class? Who will be left out, unable to afford stopping or slowing the biological aging process? If ragged old bodies count as ugly, new methods of visual rejuvenation will create an ever-widening visible divide.

*

What is the impact on our self-image to see more "beautiful faces" than ever before in the history of humankind? In 2022 the writer Eleanor Stern started a discussion on TikTok about "beauty overstimulation": social media algorithms aggressively prioritize shiny, symmetrical faces and force them on users across platforms. Users then begin to adopt the preferences of this visual economy. They are swept up by the stream of smooth, symmetrical faces, and they lend a hand in the process by embracing digital editing tools, easy-to-use filters, lighting, theatrically thick layers of makeup, and at some point, cosmetic procedures.

How overwhelmed are we by the omnipresent economy of beautiful faces? In an instance of paradoxical backlash, some social media influencers have taken it upon themselves to talk about "real" skin. Rikki Sandhu, for instance, has posted videos and close-up photos of her skin, in which she points out acne scars, chin stubble, and pores. No one looks like what is seen on screen after all, and no one should compare themselves to unrealistic, doctored images that are no longer limited to celebrities but now apply to the faces of nearly all social media users. In 2019 *New Yorker* staff writer Jia Tolentino wrote about the phantasms of digital media seeping into our ideas about the ideal face. Tolentino describes a symmetrical, youthful face with high cheekbones, catlike eyes, long lashes, a small nose, full lips, and zero pores. This face is no longer clearly white, but is instead ethnically ambiguous, potentially akin to Bella Hadid or Kim Kardashian. This generic "Instagram face" keeps transforming; it becomes an increasingly improbable sculpture, a cross between whatever wildly divergent ethnic features are especially fetishized. The face is beyond reach without cosmetic intervention. It looks like a cyborg.

Given that artificial intelligence heralds a burst in media production, we are likely to see these developments come to a head. Whereas the symmetries of antique sculpture provided the exclusive beauty ideal in the nineteenth century, today it will be an AI-generated cyborg face, symmetrical and devoid of pores, that serves as a model and vehicle for personal aspiration. In his essay "The Work of Art in the Age of Mechanical Reproduction" (1935), Walter Benjamin writes, "Man-made artifacts could always be imitated by men." This thesis fits as tidily within the logic of surgeons who fancy themselves artists imitating great works as they sculpt humans, as it does within that of modern self-optimization. Once technology permits the mass reproduction of perfection, nothing will hamper its spread. Idealized models historically were exclusive, which is what made them so coveted. The contemporary ideal, however, claims to be reproducible: with the right diet, routine, discipline, products, and treatments.

Surgery and contemporary beauty standards alike entail a conception of the human body as a sculpture and project. Benjamin writes that mechanical reproduction diminishes an artwork's aura of singularity and authenticity at the same time as it enables the spread of copies for the masses: "To an ever greater degree the work of art reproduced becomes the work of art designed for reproducibility." Benjamin thus articulates the connection between human perception and the possibilities of reproductive technologies. The further developed the technological possibilities of reproducing an ideal, the further that ideal spreads.

Although Benjamin was talking about art, the discourse about beautiful bodies allows us to apply his cultural critique to beauty standards. There are no limits to what commercial generation of images, cosmetic surgery, and AI can achieve; they can imitate any body, satisfy any ideal or fetish, and unrestrainedly produce whatever the market or state demands. The human body has material limits as well as a biological age and complex organic life, yet culturally it is increasingly seen as another object for technological reproduction. Language reveals this tendency to cast human beings as "projects" or "works in progress," like when we talk about body "hacks" or "reprogramming" ourselves—when we begin to plan, shape, and evaluate our bodies like artworks to be viewed, analyzed, and imitated. The prospect of "designer babies" with CRISPR-edited genes may represent the apex of the notion of humans as projects.

Technical reproduction decontextualizes its object, separating it from the physical and cultural locality that would make it unique. AI (re)production imitates symbols and similarities, pulls and then reassembles images from databases, without any material or biographical origin story, its genesis little more than the whim of the machine operator. Benjamin argues that even the "most perfect reproduction" cannot imitate authenticity, "its presence in time and space, its unique existence at the place where it happens to be." To bring it back to bodies: deposited in the body is the singularity of a unique human life, which is tied to place and time and bears the marks of that, with all the contradictions, all the pain, all the exhaustion, all the work. Why is our contemporary culture more interested in the blank cyborg than in humans, whose bodies bear the lines of their life story?

*

She writes to me as to a prophet:

"You opened my eyes. I see beauty in places I never did before, the beauties in the unique faces of God's children. Your message is powerful, you are a self-assured woman, and I hope my daughter turns out like you."

She writes to me as to a healer:

"I have to tell you how much you and your work have helped my sister and me appreciate our bodies. What you're doing is valuable work, giving us the strength to be beautiful. We have dark hair and stately noses. We didn't shave all summer; our eyebrows are growing in, thick and resolute. I feel amazing. Your work helps people."

She writes to me as to a scholar:

"You must know this, must have heard it before, but I am learning to love my nose, slowly but surely, because of you and your pictures. My nose isn't abnormal, for God's sake. *I* am normal. My nose doesn't need to be small and straight. It's hooked and juts out like a dagger I'm proud to wield. That's me, for God's sake. That's me. And I thank you."

She writes to me as to a muse:

"I couldn't stand myself. Then I saw your picture and put on a dress, all my hairy limbs exposed, to face the sun, so it would kiss my dark knees too."

She writes to me as to a sister:

"I see my sister in you."

He writes to me as to a stranger:

"Why is that man wearing makeup?"

I delete his comment as fast as my fingers can move, clutch my smartphone, and look around in embarrassment, as though someone might catch me red-handed. I can feel his question in my jaw and open my mouth to crack it. I don't know what I'm more ashamed of—the fact that he thought (or pretended to think) I was a man, or the fact that I immediately wanted to distance myself from the group to which he'd relegated me. Because it's not just my nose. There's more to it. There will always be something that makes them take away my femininity. In their eyes, this femininity appears as tenuous as my humanity. It's questioned the instant a body deviates from the norm by even an inch. I try to keep my cool and reorient my body toward my words, toward my images, but my jaw is clenched. I reread the other messages and try to remember who I am. A blond man sits down beside me in the subway. I pull my sleeves down over my arms, my collar up over my chin. I reread the other messages and try to remember who I am. I understand why many trans women opt for facial feminization procedures to correct so-called masculine features. Why they opt for chin recontouring, nose jobs, or jaw reduction.

I try to keep my cool and reorient my body toward my words, toward my images. I open the camera on my phone. I'm discreetly studying my chin on the screen when the man beside me sneaks a look at the display. I fish lipstick from my bag and color in my lips. He turns away. I grab his hand. I draw his fingers along my jawbone. It cuts him and he winces, pulls his hand back, and jams his bleeding fingers in his mouth. We both look down at my screen, watching the red drops trickle off the glass.

I relax my jaw, cracking it. I get up and try to keep my cool and reorient my body toward my words, toward my images. Then I roll up my sleeves and the man reaches for my arm. He nuzzles his cheek against my arm hair, closes his eyes, and sighs. I apologize for cutting him, and he apologizes for his ancestors and lets go of my arm.

H. calls as I'm getting off the train. I had sent him the title of my first exhibition, *The Drawn Angle of the Phallus Corresponds to the Angle of the Nose.*

He says, "Drawing, noses, and the phallus are all related in the title. Why is that?"

I explain to him that the title is autobiographical. Prominent noses, explicitly on women, demand space in the world, whereas the world functions according to the phallic gaze, which defines everything, the nose included.

H. hesitates, then says, "I still don't get why you're equating noses to the phallus, but maybe it's a useful contradiction."

I respond, "When my oldest sister had her nose done, I felt like someone had castrated my family. The day I made a commitment to my nose and vowed to keep it—not as a burden, but as an inheritance—was the day I reclaimed control over my image."

H. is quiet.

I continue: "I have no interest in pussy versus phallus.

Genital body politics are too limited. The hegemonic system already controls our facial features."

It sounds like H. is nodding. Something rustles, and he clears his throat. Then he says, "There's an Alexander Kluge film in which a fallen soldier's knee plays a sentient, speaking character. It reminds me of the way you treat the nose, as something constitutively beyond its usual classifications, unlike the phallus."

I tell him it's an interesting comparison and say goodbye. When I lower the smartphone from my cheek, I can feel the blond stranger's blood on my face.

III. WOLF-GIRL

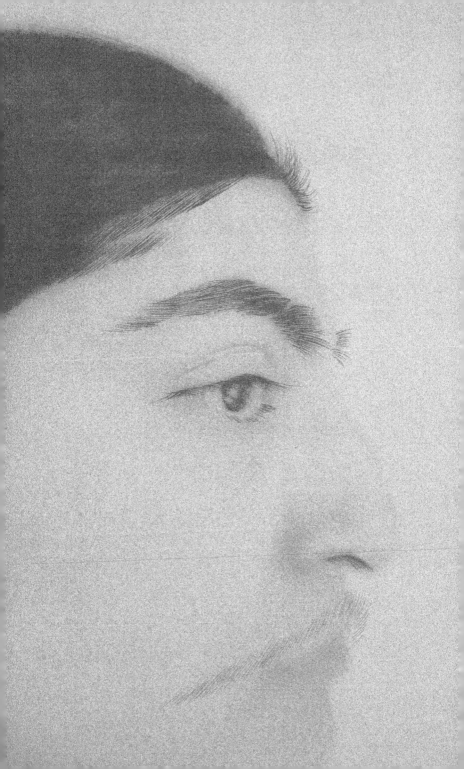

Once upon a time, a lovesick she-gorilla leaned against a tree to wallow in her loneliness. She didn't notice that the trunk was covered in a gummy substance that stuck to the hair on her arm as she leaned into it. She had no choice but to tear herself painfully away from the tree. The she-gorilla shrieked as the hair was pulled out at the roots. Her arm was now bald, and she worried that this flaw in her coat might prove repellent. Then it occurred to her that the enigmatic silverback gorilla might like it if she lost the hair entirely and had a perfectly smooth body. Week after week, the she-gorilla returned to the eucalyptus tree and removed more hair, until her limbs were fully stripped. She did not present herself to the male until after this self-sacrificing transformation, and he was thrilled, oblivious to the agonies that had led to his enjoyment. The she-gorilla continued this practice in secret. Her first baby had relatively little hair when it was born and inherited its mother's strange new sense of shame at having hair.

A gorilla recounts these evolutionary origins of hairlessness in *The Fall of Man: Or, The Loves of the Gorillas*. After encountering a deformed male gorilla, who was born nearly bald and declares that any mate of his must have even less hair, the she-gorilla uses her surprise discovery with the eucalyptus tree to begin removing her hair, and the male chooses her. This satirical piece, written from the gorillas' perspective, was the American journalist Richard Grant White's response to Charles Darwin's *The Descent of Man, and Selection in Relation to Sex*, both published in 1871. Darwin's sensational findings prompted science and media to heighten their focus on the relationship between humans and animals as the nineteenth century drew to a close.

What role has the relative hairlessness of the human body played in evolution? Were the amount and type of hair evolutionary metrics that could be used to determine how great or small the distance from the original lineage? Was sexual selection a satisfactory explanation for humans' becoming less and less hairy, more and more bare?

Questions that arose from Darwin's theory of evolution often addressed physical features that were at best useless, if not a hindrance or even deadly. One hot topic was the tendency of body hair to disappear over time. Man's exposure "to the scorching of the sun, and to sudden chills" led Darwin to expand his earlier theory of *natural* selection to include *sexual* selection. If man's relative nakedness exposes him to the elements and forces him to wear clothing—a clear disadvantage—then the reason for this development must be a sexual preference for hairless bodies. Such was Darwin's logic.

But what necessarily made naked skin so advantageous in sexual selection? Couldn't the touch of a thicketed chest be appealing, the embrace of a fuzzy body enticing? Darwin's

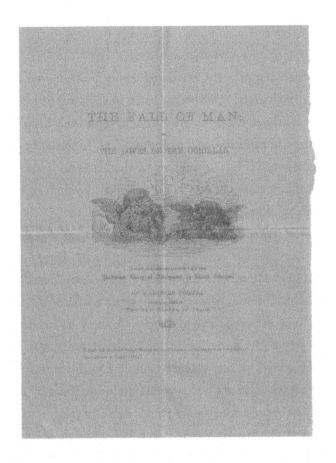

critics used the hair question as a means of discrediting him and his theory, which made it all the more important for his apostles to find evidence of the origins of man to support his reasoning. The search for a "missing link" in the evolutionary line centered on hairy humans. What was an "excessively" hairy person if not living proof of the transition from ape to Homo sapiens?

                                    *

Upon reaching puberty, the daughters of black-haired families were welcomed into the one room in their public housing project where all the women—the aunts and their daughters, the sisters and nieces—would get together. In the early afternoon, between lunch and dinner, if there was no housework to do, they gathered here. Each sat in the sunlight coming through the windows, or by a desk lamp if all the good sunny spots were taken. Each had her own 10X magnifying mirror and studied her reflection with laser focus. One of them pressed her tongue behind her upper lip, making it bulge like a hill, while another moved across the area with two threads pulled taut between fanned fingers. A third had rolled up a pant leg to the knee and sat on an open newspaper with that leg drawn in. She was watching a compilation of popular Bollywood music videos with the other women as she guided an electric epilator across her skin and tried to subdue the pain. One pass across the skin followed by three slaps on the epilated spot to swap out the searing sensation for a dull throb. The women talked, and they laughed at each other whenever someone howled. The moment the door opened, pant legs were tugged down, threads and tweezers hastily stashed. When the uncle left, after poking his head in and jokily asking what on earth was going on in here, the women returned to their conversations and the task at hand.

*

Just seven years after Darwin's book came out, a Danish physician developed a diagnostic category for excessive hairiness: hypertrichosis. The new disease sparked medical debate over the difference between pathological and normal hair growth: At what precise number of strands was a person's state considered unnatural? Unclear from the first, the line only grew murkier as racist differentiations between hair types were introduced. Despite the diagnostic question marks, hairiness—in particular visible facial hair on women—was pathologized in the medical field. One dermatologist proposed a classification system comprising six types of hair growth, each requiring a different level of treatment. The types included women with "a very fine white lanugo on the upper lip and sides of cheeks" as well as those with a "short, fine mustache." These were not cause for concern. "Coarse, stiff, long hair" growing in the same areas of a woman's face as "the male beard," however, represented a "real indication for treatment." According to this framework, men naturally had body hair, whereas women (especially young women) did not—and if they did, it was a sign of disruption or abnormality in their evolutionary development.

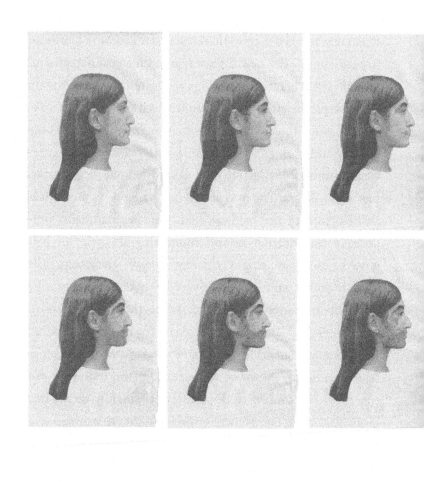

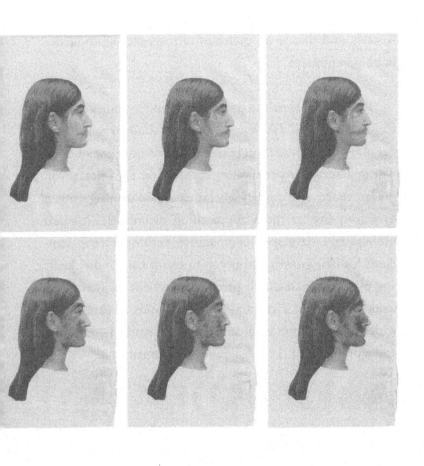

Because Darwin interpreted human hairlessness (in contrast to animals) as sexually motivated, doctors interpreted it as the central indicator of healthy sexuality in mature women, and thus as an indicator of successful reproductive pairing in humans.

Rebecca M. Herzig, a professor of gender studies at Bates College, writes in *Plucked: A History of Hair Removal* that, because of the association between fine or nonexistent body hair and sexual (reproductive) capabilities, U.S. doctors in the late nineteenth century saw little point in treating women over forty-five or those approaching menopause. Medical professionals developed comparative anthropometric standards for hair growth and began to count hairs individually and play their increasingly precise data off one another. Their work was part of a cultural shift that holds to this day, in which any deviation is understood—and studied—as illness and a problem for the development of humanity.

When I was ten, I went to see my mother's half sister, who sometimes wore a blond wig and had a habit of making snide comments about our outmoded furniture. My mom was running errands and would pick me up that evening. While my half aunt was smoking on the balcony, I arranged her leather boots alongside an upside-down glass bowl from the kitchen to serve as miniature household props as my cousin and I played Barbies. The blond dolls sat down on the boots that I had reimagined as sectional seating, and the two of us served them drinks in pistachio shells. My half aunt stubbed out her cigarette in the ashtray and picked up my leather sofa components to put them back on her feet. I didn't say anything, just watched sadly as she cleared away the play furniture. When she was done, my half aunt reached for my face and started inspecting me. "Why don't you get rid of your mustache?" she asked. "Look, we're already doing it on your cousin. This looks terrible. You're girls, you know, not boys." I responded softly that I wasn't allowed, that I was still a kid. The truth was, I had never spoken to my mother about my mustache. "Why wouldn't you be allowed? It doesn't look good. Looks like no one's taking care of you. Here, I'll do it right now." I wanted to protest, because I thought whatever she had planned for me was forbidden. Because if it weren't forbidden, wouldn't my mother have intervened already? Why would she have sent me to school looking unkempt? I mustered all my courage and tried one last time: "I'm not allowed to. I'm just a kid." But she wasn't listening. She had already slipped into the bathroom, then reappeared with a small plastic bowl of pale-blue cream. "Hold still!" She smeared the stuff on the skin above my lips, and it began to burn. I held still, in part because I thought she was about to start operating on me. I closed my eyes and inhaled the acrid chemical stench while my half aunt smoked another cigarette.

Not a Shadow of
SUPERFLUOUS
HAIR

Researchers post-Darwin considered body and facial hair secondary sexual characteristics. Degrees of hair growth were seen as indices of the "anthropological development of the race"—the further along the evolutionary development, the more pronounced the differences between men and women. Although many hypotheses in early sexology came up short, criminologists and dermatologists adopted the concepts and proposed a connection between "excessive" hair growth and "mental illness." Herzig notes that linking hairiness to insanity in the late 1800s was nothing new—one need look no further than medieval religious iconography—but that this association was now endowed with empirical scientific significance. She writes that a U.S. study from 1893, titled "Diseases of Hair: Hypertrichiasis and Mental Derangement," documented two hundred seventy-two cases of "insanity in white women"; these women had excessive facial hair that was "thicker and stiffer," like "those of the inferior races." Researchers kept looking for overlaps in the hair growth patterns of "criminally insane" and hypersexual women, whose hair was believed to indicate wildness and kinship with animals. Herzig also reflects on the fact that "transgressive women" in history were always perceived as animalistic, but that the comparison to animals took on fundamental new meaning after Darwin.

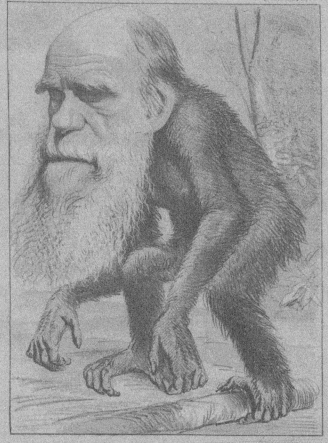

A VENERABLE ORANG-OUTANG.

A CONTRIBUTION TO UNNATURAL HISTORY.

MISSING LINK

Is it an animal?
Is it a human?
Is it an extraordinary whim of nature,
or is it the long sought-after link
between humans and apes?

Jane Goodall examines the connection between early discourse on evolution and Western performing arts in *Performance and Evolution in the Age of Darwin* (2002). The entertainment industry in the mid- to late nineteenth century saw itself as a mediator between science and the people, and it brought public attention to debates on the abnormal, exotic, and foreign. Misinterpretations of *The Descent of Man* gave rise to the theory of the "missing link" in the evolutionary line. According to these misreadings, undiscovered or "missing" links existed between modern man and his "underdeveloped" progenitors. Darwinians across disciplines took it upon themselves to ferret out this missing link and thus prove the theory of evolution once and for all. To that end, ethnological exhibitions began whetting the public's appetite for cases of deviation and difference in nature. They used the trope of the missing link to stage sensational shows and engage the audience in outrageous and shocking guessing games.

*

The demand for displaying aberrations from the norm extends back to antiquity. Non-normative bodies were similarly classified as *monsters, prodigies,* or *omens* in the Middle Ages. In *Ugliness: A Cultural History*, Gretchen E. Henderson documents a paradigm shift in people's relationship toward otherness: Religious terminology and symbols first used ugliness as a deterrent, framing it as a physical manifestation of the corrupt or condemned soul. The language and images of ugliness then changed to communicate "scientific" assumptions about what was primitive or civilized, normal or abnormal. Over the course of the seventeenth century, the notion spread of a consistent material order inherent to nature, while any irregularities represented not heavenly miracles but earthly anomalies. Darwinism, however, sparked the systematic and collective scientific search for deviance.

In *Staging Stigma: A Critical Examination of the American Freak Show*, the theater studies scholar Michael M. Chemers argues that Darwin's analytical rhetoric fed straight into the popular genre of adventure tales. These romantic narratives expanded on scientific debates about human genealogy and rendered them imperialist fantasies of conquest, discovery, progress, and civilization. The notion of shared origins—albeit with their own ideas of culture and nature as paramount—enabled white colonists to cast themselves as the heroes of human history and everyone else as regressive and deviant.

In museums now tailored to the masses, ordinary people could marvel at *freaks* or *wonders of nature* with their own eyes and draw their own conclusions. Such exhibitions allowed the general public to playact as scientists and speculate about the origins and significance of the subjects on display. These spaces provided a voyeuristic service by bringing elite scientific discourse to the middle class, all at the expense of the people on display. P. T. Barnum, father of the American circus and sideshow of *human curiosities*, was only a year Darwin's junior. As part of the greater debate about evolution and man's origins, Barnum's advertising copy read, "They are not freaks or monstrosities but the incredible results of fundamental continuous natural laws." Chemers uses Barnum—the Greatest Showman—to illustrate how freak discourse needed Darwinism to imbue it with gravitas, while Darwinism needed the freak show to reach the middle class and thus the so-called masses. Audiences included doctors and scientists, who recounted the fascinating cases they encountered there in publications and memoirs. Several outfits even commissioned such texts to lend their marketing materials legitimacy. Though they spun exotic biographies for their "freaks," these shows leaned linguistically on the scientific authority of ethnology.

The bioethicist Rosemarie Garland-Thomson describes how the display of unusual bodies followed ritualized forms of viewing in her essay "Making Freaks: Visual Rhetorics and the Spectacle of Julia Pastrana": by showcasing bodies that transgressed the supposed boundaries between human and animal or man and woman, organizers provoked a confusion of categories. Spectators were ready to pay for the discomfort and delight they came to expect. The challenge facing freak shows was to choreograph *appeal* and *repulsion* in such a way that left "civilized" middle-class audiences feeling secure in their sense of self, not overly rattled. Visitors gaping at human exhibits did not feel boorish, barbaric, or mean; instead, because of freak shows' scientifically inflected language, they regarded their experiences as educational, their own voyeurism a commendable interest in the natural sciences.

*

A woman dressed in clothing foreign to her native culture stares wide-eyed into space, her newborn beside her. Two men stand nearby. They gaze theatrically at mother and child to make absolutely clear what they're doing. One is in a pinstripe suit and tie with a blond mop top hairstyle and beard. The other has his hair combed back and wears a turtleneck and square glasses with thick black frames. The men behold the mother and her child with hammed-up expressions of shock, while the mother and child stare into nothingness from the glass eyes that have been planted in their dead bodies. It's January of 1970 in Malmö, Sweden, and two white men are staring at the embalmed corpses of Julia Pastrana and her baby.

Given its staged quality, the photo—presumably an advertisement for the exhibited bodies—comes across as laughable and grotesque. Looking at it, there are long moments when it's easy to think that the eager observers are harassing nothing more than mannequins, but Pastrana's dead body and that of her son were publicly displayed in museums, circuses, and amusement parks for well over a hundred years. At some point after this image was captured, their preserved remains were stored in the basement of a forensic institute in Oslo, where they remained available to researchers. Finally, in 2013, after more than ten years of public petitioning and more than a century and a half after her death, Pastrana was granted a proper burial near her birthplace in Sinaloa, Mexico.

In *Ugliness: A Cultural History*, Henderson reflects on how difficult it is to tell the stories of those bodies exhibited as so-called freaks. How can we talk about them without our words putting them back on display? During her lifetime and posthumously, Pastrana was referred to as the "ugliest woman in the world," but when Norway decided to repatriate her remains to Mexico, the presiding committee at least made an attempt at critical interpretation:

> The attention Julia Pastrana received while alive, and particularly the treatment of her remains after her death, has to a great extent consisted of various forms of interest in her particular appearance, a fascination which has sometimes been not only ethically unacceptable, but grotesque.

Henderson comments that in retrospect, the committee declared Pastrana's exhibitors and spectators—and not her—grotesque, and thus ugly.

The gaze has turned: it is not those who are looked at who are ugly, but those who look with the intention to dehumanize. How do we look back at *deviant bodies*—what fuels our interest in looking at these bodies? Should we not look at all? Has the time come to avert our gaze and turn it on ourselves? Whichever way we turn, whose gaze are we adopting? Whose tradition defines the way we see? Whose stance do we take, and whose side are we on when we look at people like Pastrana?

*

In "Making Freaks," Garland-Thomson unpacks the visual norms that influenced interpretations of Pastrana's body. The bioethicist reads contemporary medical, ethnological, and commercial texts about Pastrana's case in a retroactive effort to understand the ideological goals behind exhibiting her—and thus the role of people with disabilities in our cultural narratives. Garland-Thomson uses an approach from disability studies that reads the label *disability* not as inferiority but as a cultural system that stigmatizes the possibility of "human variation." Ergo: Pastrana may have been physically different from most people, because of her enlarged jaw and the thick hair on her body, but these deviations from the expectations of human appearance did not lead to the life Pastrana was forced to have. Her life as a "freak" was not forced upon her by her body, but by humans.

Pastrana belonged to an indigenous group living in Mexico's Sierra Madre range. As a child, she was kidnapped by the governor of Sinaloa, who took her home as a human curiosity. By her early twenties, she was advertised as a sensation of the stage and "wonder of the world" and sent on tour to major Western cities. Many human exhibits at the time, including Pastrana, were controlled by managers who reaped the profits. Her manager and "husband," Theodore Lent, remarried after Pastrana's death; his second wife had similar features and was forced to play Pastrana's younger sister, allowing Lent to continue to exploit the Pastrana brand. Even the earnings from exhibits of Pastrana's dead body went to this man. He packaged Pastrana as a "marvelous anomaly" who could dance, sing, and converse in English and Spanish like "civilized people" in European dress, unlike other members of her tribe, who were denigrated as "ordinary savages."

Garland-Thomson juxtaposes the voyeuristic exploitation of "freaks" with clinical diagnoses of illness: modern medical discourse describes Pastrana's distinctive features as forms of hypertrichosis and hyperplasia. Ultimately, these terms ("elite, specialized jargon," as Garland-Thomson puts it) amount to little more than categories that again reduce

Pastrana to a body, only this time it's an *abnormality* in the pages of medical journals, rather than on the stage. We never really allow divergent bodies to play a role in our cultural narratives without subjecting them to stigma.

A CHRONOLOGY OF HAIRINESS

It's the summer of 1999, and my mother smiles at the sight of me seated on the back of a pony. It carries me around in a circle. A German woman pets the animal. For a second, though, I believe I'm the one being petted. Her hand grazes my hairy leg.

It's the fall of 2004, and I'm taking the bus home. A little German girl, younger and littler than I am, asks her mother in a loud voice, "Why does that girl have a beard?" I'm sitting across from them, and I lower my gaze and dash out at the next stop.

It's the summer of 2006, and I'm in shorts with shaved legs, sitting in a paddleboat with A. at Hamburg Stadtpark. A., that towheaded boy with pale white skin and icy blue eyes, looks at my thighs. "What are those black dots you have there?" I lower my gaze and count the dark roots that glow through my skin.

It's the summer of 2008, and E.—who once claimed to be related to the soccer player Gerald Asamoah—snaps at me during a fight: "You have hair in your nose." I respond, "So do you." He says, yeah, but he's a guy.

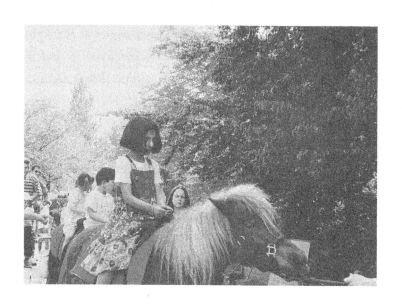

It's the summer of 2018, and two days in a row, independently of each other, two journalist friends of mine reach out and stroke the thick, dark hair on my arms without asking. Both recall, "I used to have hair like this on my arms, maybe even more than you."

*

In *Plucked*, Herzig cites a wide range of twentieth-century medical literature, which documented one dramatic case after another: patients were experiencing terrible depression; they were isolating themselves; they were disgusted by the sight of themselves; they hated themselves; they wished they didn't exist . . . they could not endure the hair on their bodies, anywhere from the hairline down. They were melancholy, embittered, and wanted to die to escape their embarrassment.

Women who hope to marry are frantic, because their skin is being read. One can tell from their legs what they think about declining birth rates; folks take one look at their armpits to learn their stance on the use of military force; and what appears to be a screed against domestic violence is inscribed on their upper lip. The body covered in hair is increasingly a body covered in script.

Herzig describes how the renegotiation of gender roles in the West has amplified accusations of masculinization. A woman who advocates for her rights and independence is masculinized, and the public is starting to derive the *modern woman's* degree of masculinization from her hair growth. Herzig provides examples of doctors searching for hairy connections among lesbians, businesswomen, and activists.

A woman who hoped to marry—one who wished to distinguish herself from society's leftist, *foreign*, or *queer* antagonists—was not allowed to have body hair. Herzig teases out the ways in which political aversion toward rule-breaking women overlaps with implicitly racist biases about hygiene and health.

Visual distance was sought from rule-breakers generally, as well as from non-white immigrants, who were perceived as impure, dirty, uncivilized, and alien.

The first issue of *Ms.* magazine, published in 1972, features an article titled "Body Hair: The Last Frontier." The piece addresses the role of body hair in the feminist fight, authors Harriet Lyons and Rebecca Rosenblatt examining how social pressure to shave one's armpits, legs, and pubic area kept women from experiencing their bodies fully. Constant shaving and the obsession with replicating the smooth skin of an innocent "little girl" was yet another perpetual task that kept women occupied. In the parlance of second-wave feminism, the authors call for women to appreciate the real appearance and aromas of their bodies.

In her cultural history of hair removal, Herzig includes an anecdote Lyons and Rosenblatt use to illustrate the stigma against hairy women: a young woman is involved in a cycling accident, and as a member of the New York Police Department inspects her injured, unshaven leg, he asks, "You're not Puerto Rican, are you?" The stigma the white feminist writers at *Ms.* were trying to highlight was the association between body hair and "dirty foreigners," and presumably their feminist goal was to fight that association. Not all unshaven women are dirty or foreigners or dirty foreigners.

*

TikTok: "My daughter has hairy arms,
should I just do it before she starts middle school?
She's in fifth grade and so far no one has made
fun of her arms."

M. is in elementary school. Her name begins like mine, but she's someone else's daughter; I could be her aunt. She goes to school every morning with a gray shadow across her mouth. Later, she trembles with shame in the locker room, where she and the other girls in her class have to bare their legs. Hers are silver in the fluorescent light. No one notices, until someone does, and M. can sense their eyes on her soft legs. She folds her jacket like a curtain and, standing at the far end of the room, drapes it between herself and the others. Even at a distance she can hear them whispering behind their hands. "Like a monkey," one of them mouths, words that M. can read between the white fingers.

*

M. hadn't yet decided if she was a feminist.
M. didn't yet have any armpit hair that could do the talking
for her.
M. wore pants in summer.
M. observed the golden shimmer
on other girls' legs.
M. observed that they only shaved
up to their knees,
and that everything above their knees shimmered like gold.

I could never love a man
with less hair on his body
than I allow to grow
on my cheeks
on my back
all down my arms

Is that so?—he asks, his arm
resting on mine
Both could be his arms
They're his if he wants
They're yours if you want
I respond, my arm
resting on his

Our arms entangled
we softly brush
lost eyelashes from each other's face
He takes a finger
and traces a word
on my back for me
He takes a finger
and brushes my shameful strands
aside for me, like curtains
He takes a finger
and traces a word for me.

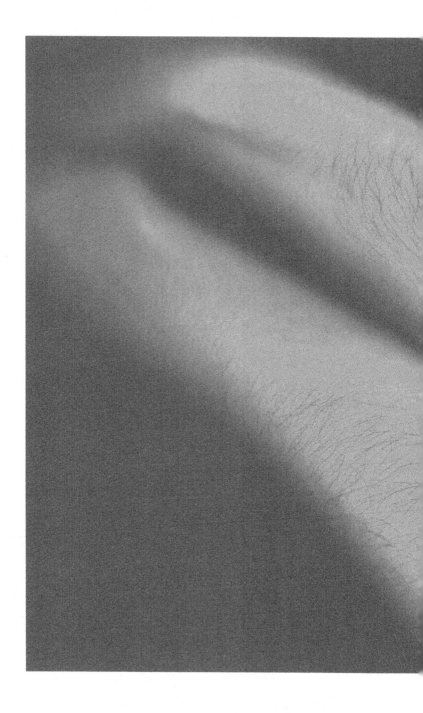

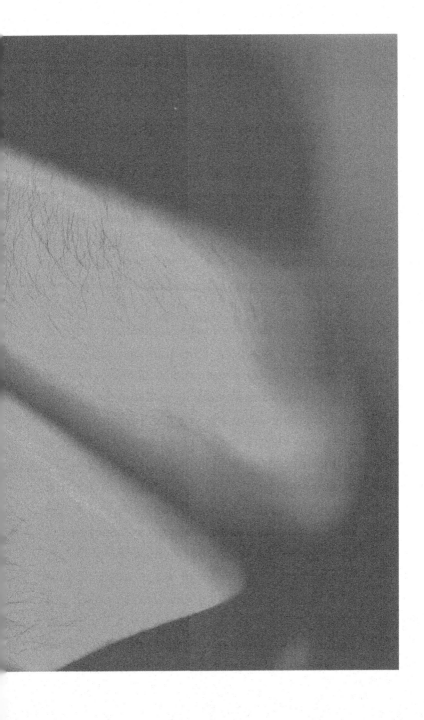

A WOMAN EXPOSED

An army of little black hairs pushes through the white powder, a floury coating on sweaty skin, the wheat hue of which is revealed in the hand. She keeps brushing the same hair from her face, and every time her hand rises, the contrast shows who she really is under the veneer. Afghan retailers imported the powder from South Korea. "Why don't you wear makeup closer to your skin color?" I ask, baffled. I'm fourteen and don't wear any makeup at all.

On our trip to Kabul, my cousins accidentally swapped my suitcase with a stranger's. I then accidentally got off the train with the suitcase and even accidentally flew on with this unknown woman's clothing to Kabul for a different cousin's wedding. Soon after we got there, we headed to one of Kabul's biggest, newest malls, located in Shahr-e Naw, an upscale neighborhood in the heart of the city. The towering shopping center held one perfumery after the next, interspersed with gold dealers and jewelers, bridal shops, and boutiques selling fancy apparel as flamboyant as their names: Luxury Palace, Prestige Fashion, Royal Deluxe Boutique, Diamond Beauty. In an act of aesthetic protest, and in an attempt to draw a line between myself and Kabul's kitsch and pathos, all I bought was a minimalist knee-length dress with matching beige linen-cotton-blend pants. It was a two-piece set my cousins here in Afghanistan might have worn to do chores, but never to an occasion as celebratory as a wedding.

My white-powdered cousin turns to me in astonishment and responds in a wounded tone:

"You all expose your skin to feel pretty. All we have is our faces."

Embarrassed, I clasp one of my shoulders, which protrudes from my sleeveless dress. This bare shoulder didn't come cheap either. Only a year earlier, our mother still insisted on sewing four-inch sleeves onto every sleeveless dress of mine or my sisters' as a compromise, the result of yearslong discussion about the meaning of bare shoulders and the view of our armpits. Before my sisters and I succeeded in abolishing these sleeves, I would roll them up as high as the girth of my arms would allow. My bare skin began at the shoulder, my cousin's at her face.

*

Gillette is the Razor of the Great War. A World War against body hair. Gillette had produced disposable razors since 1908, but it wasn't until World War I, when the U.S. military began requiring soldiers on active duty to shave themselves, that the company booked record sales.

Gillette introduced the first razor for women in 1915, but the new consumer base would need a lot of cajoling before shaving really took off. Well into the twentieth century, running water, mass-produced mirrors, and private bathrooms were rare. Industry and infrastructure required further development to open the doors for female shaving and to make the work of hair removal personal, affordable, and something the female masses could do in private. Morals, too, were in want of change: the 1920s saw a shift in Western women's fashion toward showing more skin, a moment that could be referred to as the Great Exposure of the female body. Newly exposed, unshaven female underarms provided a market that razor blade manufacturers like Gillette could tap. Companies placed more and more ads in women's magazines to generate the need as well as the social pressure to shave—smooth underarms and legs became a matter of hygiene, class, and femininity in these campaigns. Herzig writes that a turning point in cementing the regular practice of shaving came in the 1940s, when World War II limited production of nylon stockings, meaning women had to put their bare legs on display every day. More skin followed, more visibility, more marketable area for the growth of the cosmetics industry.

*

Talking to a friend, I admitted my hesitation toward watching her film about hammams. Since their first portrayals in European art history, hammams—as well as any realm of thought about the bodies of Muslim women—have served as objects of Orientalization and the male gaze. I couldn't imagine how that space and the nude bodies it holds could be presented without vestigial associations with eroticism and exoticism. When I finally watched *Shedding Skin* by Yumna Al-Arashi, I was deeply affected. The film moved and touched places I hadn't known existed in me. The naked, wet bodies on screen were familiar to me, not foreign. They exuded love and ease; they weren't erotic. The way old and young bodies washed each other reminded me of my mother washing my grandmother, my sisters and me washing our mother. What I saw—naked bodies bathing together—was vulnerable and intimate. I was wondering how my friend captured these images, when suddenly I spotted her there among the women. My gaze swept over their bodies casually, as if I were there with them too. Just one small detail caused my gaze to linger: the sight of tiny black hairs encircling a female nipple.

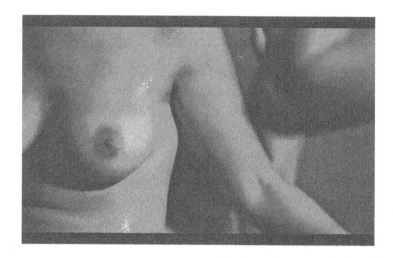

An unpracticed hand repeatedly shaving over the same patch of skin can result in wounds and inflammation. When you shave the thin, sensitive skin of the inner thigh, the hair grows back within forty-eight hours. Prickly stubble chafes and pokes, itches and scratches. It's too short, though, barely enough there to shave again. Nevertheless, I would, though the blades cut less hair than they did skin. Little gashes bleeding down my legs every time.

*

She described the contortions she performed, how she'd wrench herself around to shave her own back, until one day a friend climbed into the bathtub with her. Her friend took the razor, soaped up her small back, and drew the blade in vertical lines along her body until all the lather and all the hair was gone, until the only hair left was the hair on her head, her eyebrows, and lashes.

They always return, as though they were hers, as though she were theirs. She always finds herself back at the drain, watching them drown. Then they poke back out of her exhausted skin, as they always do. E. cries into her father's lap. He dries the salty trails down her cheeks. *My beautiful girl, don't cry. Every rose has its thorns.*

*

It's 2003, just two years after the U.S. invasion and the end of the first authoritarian Taliban regime in Afghanistan. A blond woman haggles with a young man in a stall in Kabul. With the documentarian Liz Mermin's camera rolling, the woman explains that she's a hairdresser from New York who founded a program "to open the beauty school for the women," an initiative underwritten by the giants of the U.S. fashion industry. The six hundred afghani he was charging would equal about six dollars for the American, but by this point she is thronged by curious passersby, and the camera captures the impassive young shopkeeper dropping his price to five hundred afghani.

He reminds her in parting that Afghanistan has been at war for the last twenty years, to which she responds, "That's why we're here, to help." The blond beautician works for Beauty Without Borders, an American nongovernmental organization made possible by "development aid" and cooperation among the fashion and beauty industries, U.S. military, and newly created Afghan Ministry of Women's Affairs. The famed *Vogue* editor-in-chief Anna Wintour's support was allegedly decisive in securing the project's financing. In her article "The Biopower of Beauty: Humanitarian Imperialisms and Global Feminisms in an Age of Terror," the cultural scholar Mimi Thi Nguyen describes how the initiative viewed itself as providing a form of idealistic humanitarian aid that helped people help themselves. There was also the convenient allusion to Doctors Without Borders and the medical aid it provides, with this initiative providing a *universal beauty* "without borders" exported by means of a training program for hairstylists and makeup artists. The women and their beauty salons were meant to serve as an "oasis amid the ugliness of war," Nguyen writes.

Beauty Without Borders wasn't "just about providing lipstick," project director Patricia O'Connor insisted in an interview with ABC News. "It's about restoring self-esteem and independence." Another cosmetician, Deborah Rodriguez—who would later write a best-selling book, *Kabul Beauty School*, as well as novels including *The Zanzibar Wife* and *The Moroccan Daughter*—opens her classes with similarly preachy language about her notions of beauty. In Mermin's

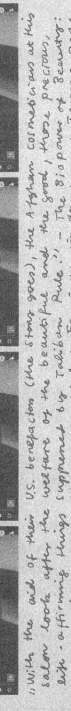

Everywoman - Latvian Dads and Kabul Beauty Salon

We used burqas to cover our rollers...

...and the Taliban would say,
'Why is your burqa so high?'

They would beat us with
a leather strap.

Funny days.

["By Afghan standards, Americans wore so little makeup that we looked pretty much like men - and homely men at that," Ms. Rodriguez wrote.] Exit and 200? Review—New York Times conceding defeat on that front.] on William Grimes on "Kabul Beauty School" by Deborah Rodriguez

"With the aid of their U.S. benefactors (the story goes), the Afghan cosmeticians at his salon look after the welfare of the beautiful and the good, those precious, life-affirming things suppressed by Taliban Rule." - The Biopower of Beauty: Humanitarian Imperialisms and Global Feminism in an Age of Terror. 2011. in: SIGNS, Vol. 36, No. 2 pp. 359-383, by Minoo Iraji Nguyen

2004 film *The Beauty Academy of Kabul*, we see Rodriguez admonishing Afghan women to remember the connection between their appearance and the future of their country: how could Afghanistan be expected to change and develop a modern look if the women didn't change, themselves?

In an Australian news feature on the school, we meet Wajma, who is enrolled in the program along with her aunt Jamila. She is doing the training, she says, because given growing demand, beauticians earn more than doctors in Kabul. Like many of her classmates—single mothers, widows, or women whose husbands are sick or out of work—Wajma is the breadwinner and hopes to open her own salon. The beauty business is booming, after all. In preparation for that future, trainees are given practical guideposts: How long should different cosmetic chemicals be left on? How much makeup does a *modern* woman wear?

Nguyen argues that the promise of beauty as freedom coincided with the United States' imperialist war. What exactly was the beauty school promising if its promises were linked both structurally and ideologically to military objectives and the destruction of Afghanistan? While the Americans coordinated drone strikes elsewhere in the country, U.S. Army officials guarded the Beauty Without Borders graduation ceremony. The ethnologist Julie Billaud writes in *Kabul Carnival: Gender Politics in Postwar Afghanistan* that Beauty Without Borders was one of many projects from that period with the shared goal of creating the "new Afghan woman," to show the world that Afghanistan had the capacity for being *civilized* and *modern*. In so-called developing nations, Billaud explains, projects like these were as common as participation in international beauty pageants, the countries' aim being to demonstrate to a global audience how *progressive* and *liberal* they were by showcasing their women. In the case of the American beauty academy, however, the Afghan Ministry of Women's Affairs retracted its support after only a year. Its cooperation with the Western project was compromising its own fight for women's rights. Billaud cites the Afghan press and relates how growing criticism of the U.S. occupation was also changing the perception of liberal body practices among Afghan women. The ways women styled their hair and how much skin they exposed were interpreted as the direct result of foreign influence and women's corruption by the occupiers. Kabul Beauty School failed because the *beauty* it sought to import is not, in fact, universal (though organizers claimed otherwise) but imperial; as such, it does not exist without borders (as those same organizers hoped) but as part of a military front—a front that advances on the bodies of Afghan women by way of white face powder and a hem exposing a bare shoulder.

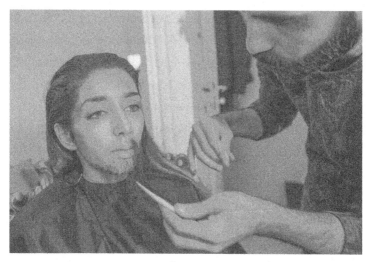

Forough Alaei, from the 2019 photo series "Crying for Freedom" showing a makeup artist applying a fake beard to a woman because female spectators in Iran are banned from attending stadium soccer matches.

My mother falls three times. Twice she breaks her leg; the other time it's a rib. We take her to the doctor who discovers a hole in my mother's eardrum. It looks like an old injury that never healed and has now become inflamed, throwing her off-balance. *Did you injure your ear a long time ago, many years ago?* I translate. My mother tries to recall, then responds with a nod, which her doctor notes with a second nod. What kind of injury was it? *Someone slapped me,* she says on our way home following the appointment. How brutal was that blow? Who raised their hand against my mother? Whose loathsome hand? I know it wasn't my father, because my mother is always saying her husband never laid a finger on her. It's a story meant to distinguish him, because the very absence of violence is praiseworthy in the world my mother grew up in. Who was it, then, who had beaten her about the head so badly that decades later, the injury to her ear was making her fall and break her bones? My mother reluctantly admits it was her brother. She makes me promise he won't ever learn what came of his striking her. He would never forgive himself. That impulsive young man back then—he was only trying to protect her, my mother says. With her first-ever paycheck from her job as an elementary school teacher, she had bought tickets to a buzkashi match. She and a friend attended the equestrian game, in which twenty-odd men on horseback compete for a goat carcass. My mother had a great day and cheerfully returned home after nightfall. Her brother was waiting for her, consumed with rage, unable to comprehend how his grown sister could have allowed herself such autonomy. That's it, that's the story behind his hitting her. It was a blow that was now making my mother stagger, trip, and fall. Twenty years after he hit her, the man with the imprint of her injuries on his hand storms unseen into our living room in Hamburg:

"I need to have a word with you, sister. Your daughter is dragging our family into ruin. She is unmarried, yet goes around looking like someone's wife. She's showing off for men, not acting her age. If she starts plucking her eyebrows today, tomorrow it will be my daughters reaching for the tweezers. They're disfiguring their innocent faces into the faces of wanton women. We can't allow it. Tell your daughter to leave her eyebrows be. Tell her she has to listen."

His hand wavers from my mother's ear to my sister's brows. I try to imagine my mother grabbing his wrist and breaking it in two, but his wrist goes untouched. My mother politely keeps quiet, and my sister's brows get thinner and thinner, until they resemble two pale threads. They change shape and grin at my uncle like splayed legs. They thrash about and send us into welcome ruin. My ears and eyebrows remain untouched.

IV. THE UNDEAD

In 1962 the Iranian poet Forugh Farrokhzad shot *The House Is Black*, her celebrated first and only film. The lyrical twenty-minute documentary opens with a warning that viewers are about to witness a depiction of ugliness, a show of sorrow that no feeling person should ignore. This introduction establishes the film's framework by acknowledging the ugliness of the coming images and at the same time exposing viewers to them since the exclusion and visual erasure of ugliness were in part responsible for the suffering portrayed. Farrokhzad then shows disturbing and touching shots of people in an Iranian leper colony reading passages from the Old Testament and Quran about the beauty of God's creations. Children whose faces appear melted, whose hands are reduced to stubs, recite verses of thanks for having been created by God, for His having given them ears, eyes, and hands that allow them to experience the beauty of the world. The incongruity grows harder and harder to bear until Farrokhzad's voice asks:

"Who is this in hell praising you, Oh Lord?"

The film was commissioned by Iran's Society for Assisting Lepers and produced by Golestan Films, a studio financed by the National Iranian Oil Company. Its focus is a leper colony founded just two years earlier with support from Farah Pahlavi, the wife of the shah. The official mandate of the project—namely, to teach audiences about leprosy and its treatment—did not stop the poet from expressing empathetic criticism: if leprosy is not uncurable—twice the filmmaker repeats "not incurable"—the film implicitly asks why we are seeing these wasted bodies banished like pariahs to a remote colony. The accusation is written all over the faces peering into the camera.

Drugs to halt the disease from advancing have existed since 1948, and later, antibiotics were developed that contribute to its cure. The film depicts daily life in the colony, providing insight into medical treatment, schooling, and a wedding. We see children playing; we see one woman combing her hair and another applying makeup to what is left of her eyes. Life could go on for these people, if someone took care of them.

In an interview twenty-five years after *The House Is Black* was made, Ebrahim Golestan—Farrokhzad's partner and the film's producer—revealed that the piece was an allegory of Iranian society, which had been confined and made sick by the monarchy. To that end, Farrokhzad's poems convey her own loneliness and grief in the film. In her analysis "Women in Window," the film scholar Nicole Brenez argues that Farrokhzad expands the form of objective documentation into a complex mental image that condenses the lives on screen, her own words, and the political context. At the end of the film we see a boy with leprosy at school, and the film suggests that everything depicted there could be a product of his imagination: We see him prompted to compose a sentence with the word *house*. He thinks about it, and we join him in seeing before his mind's eye the entire population of the colony moving toward the camera, just as the gate to the compound closes on them. Then the boy writes the film title in white chalk on the blackboard, "The house is black." In a way, though, the film was produced "by leprosy as much as against it," Brenez observes. The film would not exist without the lepers' experiences, but it was also made to put an end to these experiences, not just report on them. It's not about a "subjective appropriation of the condition of the sick by a compassionate poetess"—Farrokhzad was not looking simply to create reportage; she made an effort to grant the lepers agency. The filmed bodies are the source of their own representation, Brenez continues, which makes them the owners of this representation; first and foremost, the film is for them.

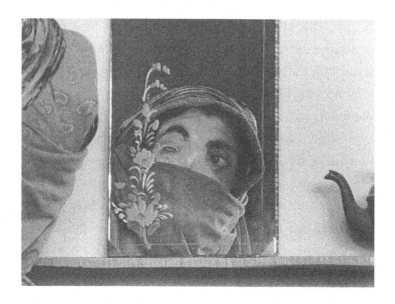

To feel empathy we must somehow find a way to put ourselves mentally in someone else's place. Though a mental image will never approximate the torment experienced by lepers, still there's an attempt at empathy, the one and only way to start seeing with care. Farrokhzad's images collapse the distance between the screen and our gaze. We watch as others watch us apathetically observe their plight. Having our gaze returned becomes unbearable and denies us the option of disinterest. The documentary does not allow for pathologizing, despite its focus on illness. We see people with no choice but to live in diseased bodies, something for which they are banished from their homes and locked up. We cannot rid ourselves of the sight of the lepers. Their visible disfigurement and helpless humility despite their forced exclusion make us aware of our own humanity, mortality, and responsibility. In *Illness as Metaphor*, Susan Sontag warns against the figurative use of illness. Illness is neither a mythological state of being nor a moral failure, Sontag writes; illness should be viewed as illness, not as a sign. Brenez praises *The House Is Black* for avoiding the pitfall of being so overwhelmed by suffering that a sense of powerlessness in the film transfigures or canonizes the sufferers. *The House Is Black* holds steady in its poetic candor: We see people engaged in the daily work of survival, nothing more and nothing less. The indictment takes aim at everyone everywhere else: Why must their daily survival be so difficult?

*

How to look at illness, then? If our ideas of ugliness are in large part informed by the sick and suffering body, how best to approach this body? What might it look and feel like— this view and approach—without ugliness? How to see ugliness without mystifying or blocking it out?

In the early twentieth century, doctors in Europe pushed for the systematic isolation of lepers, to allow the disease to die out with them. Leprosy had to be reported in many places; in Greece, for instance, a law crafted with the help of a German leprosy specialist required that all lepers be deported to select locations. Epaminondas Remoundakis, a

law student, fell ill with leprosy in 1936 and was interned
for twenty years on the Cretan island of Spinalonga, which
was a leper colony from 1903 to 1957. His entire life, he
advocated for the rights of lepers, in whose company he had
spent so many years on the island. The French ethnographer
Maurice Born published an account of Remoundakis's recol-
lections in *Vies et morts d'un Crétois lépreux* (Lives and Deaths
of a Cretan Leper). In the 1972 interview that informed the
book, Remoundakis shares his memories of the colony. He
recalls an inflection point, when at a doctor's appointment he
was asked to unbutton his sleeves and roll them up. A long
time passed before he realized that the act of unbuttoning
his shirtsleeves signified the "rupture of his life," a "severance
from other humans," the "passage to the other side of the
river, never to return."

Remoundakis detected the first signs of leprosy as a child,
but he managed to keep the illness a secret and even enroll in
law school, until relatives informed the police. He recounts
his arrest and deprivation of rights, which persisted year after
year in utter disregard of medical advances. He always wondered why he had been condemned, why he had been banished, what his crime was. The sick were left to their own
devices on the small island; there were no trained caregiv-
ers and scarcely any medication. Remoundakis fought for
improved living conditions on Spinalonga, whereas many
others hoped in vain that their stint in the colony was tem-
porary. Remoundakis advocated for the construction of

footpaths, a school—at which he then taught—and a café as a gathering place. He tells Born that doctors, officials, even filmmakers would visit the island as if it were a zoo, and each time, residents hoped for improvements that never came: "To this day, they have unfortunately all betrayed us. None gave us what we wanted or what they had promised to show the world." Years later, Born added the subtitle *Archéologie d'une arrogance* (Archaeology of an Arrogance) to the book he and Remoundakis had coauthored. In some ways, the arrogance of the outside world of the hale, which hurt Remoundakis and the other lepers—ruined their lives—was more uncompromising than the disease itself. What could a caring view of illness and suffering even look like, without losing ourselves in the sensationalized rhetoric of ugliness and the exclusionary language of pathology? Remoundakis answers this question in the book:

"Some made a show of compassion,
others of revulsion,
but we did not want them
to hate
or pity us.
All we needed was love."

UNSIGHTLY

We don't want to be ugly—not when we're dying, and not even when we're dead.

She describes one of her fears to me. She imagines being so busy and worn out, she doesn't get around to shaving, first for a week, then several. Her legs and thighs, her calves, the skin on her back, belly, and crotch become covered in hair that she would otherwise routinely remove. She tells herself she'll take care of it once she has time, once exams are over, once she's met all her deadlines. No one will see her till then; no one will touch her. She alone observes the way her skin fills up and darkens; the way her hand moves over the hair; the way the stubble pokes through her black tights; the way it springs from her underpants like the crown of a tree on her lower back when she bends over, until her hand pulls her shirt down to cover the bare skin. She doesn't want to stretch, either forward or backward, so as not to reveal the growth on her skin. These moments are secret; they exist only between her and her body. The morning before her last exam, she's rushing out the door and across the street when a car hits her. She lies on the ground. Strangers come to her aid; the ambulance arrives. Paramedics gather round, cut her bloodied pants and lift her blood-soaked shirt. Curious bystanders see her hairy belly and make faces. That's her worst nightmare. Because a hairy death like that is so much more frightening than an unhairy one, she feels compelled to keep up with hair removal forever. She's made a pact with her sister. Should she ever find herself incapable of shaving, her sister would step in. And she would shave her sister, if she were in that position. The sisters would visit each other in the hospital, the healthy sister shaving the paralyzed or comatose sister to preserve her dignity. The sisters promised themselves: we will shave—or be shaved—until we die.

*

We fear ugliness. We see it in the infirmity and decline of aging and sick bodies, a helplessness that threatens to rob us of our vanity, pride, and dignity. How much say do we have in our appearance when it's others tending, touching, seeing our bodies? Losing control over when and how we are seen means losing autonomy and command over ourselves. Illness and old age erode that command, that possibility of choice in what to show and what to hide. In illness and old age, our bodies begin to betray us. The worst betrayal is when death relinquishes our bodies, now unavailable to us, wholly to others.

We're afraid of ugliness, afraid of finding it in old people's wrinkles, in the scars, sores, wounds, lumps, deformities, fluids, and fractures of those we see approaching death. By forever banishing the frail and ailing from our sight, we ourselves hope for refuge from the ever-present threat of death. The frail and ailing are repellent to us, so that by distancing ourselves from them, we may forget that mortality even exists.

My God,
my God,
why did you forsake me!

DYING PRAYER

The German-born American sculptor Kiki Smith shifted her focus to human mortality—as expressed in the feeble and maltreated body—after first her father died, then her sister.

Nothing will ever undo what we discover in encountering the sheer vulnerability of the human body in the form of the sheer vulnerability of a body we love and respect. It stays with us forever. Illness and injury are so destructive and cruel, and leave us so exposed, they have the power to rob us of shame and autonomy. Until one day, our own death demands the surrender of our body and hands it off to others, as though it had never belonged to us.

Do you really not belong to me, dear body?

Smith cannot escape the sight of her dying ones. She scrutinizes the shame we feel when someone else's death reminds us of our own mortality, and we can't help but see it in others. Her pieces about bodies that can no longer be controlled, such as her sculpture of a woman crawling on all fours, trailing shit behind her—these artworks stare us down. We don't want to look, but they cast such a penetrating gaze at us that our insides are turned out, exposed for all to see.

Why are you so far
from my cries and pleas, my screams,
my silence!
My God!
I scream! when it's light out, and you do not hear;
when it's dark, and you do not answer.

If *ugly* means being old, ill, and unloved, it's not really that
   we hate the ugly; it's that we fear our own mortality,
   fragility, and loneliness.

When my mother was slowly dying,
her body was old and ill,
but she was not unloved. She was loved, forever.

How could I call my dying mother
ugly, though what remained of her body
at the end frightened me.

I kissed her dear hand with its mole
and the hennaed half-moon
that had survived on the tip of her nail.

We kissed her hands and cheeks
to provide her dying body solace.
There were days when the people who wanted to kiss and
   love her
were packed in so tight,
it allowed me to forget
that this was the ugliest moment of my life.

If we are to believe that *ugly* means unsightly,
repellent, hateful,
then certainly her illness was those things; her illness was hated.
We hated it like a punishment, like a flood
claiming our home.

We stood close together,
our faces tearstained and hands trembling,
but did we hate the body
illness had befallen?

There is nothing ugly about the sight of a beloved person
losing their body to illness:
the sight of a ruin, when we know
what is buried within,
behind,
under,
out in front of the rubble.

Ugliness is repulsive no longer
when it touches us,
comes up close
and enfolds us.
When it falls to pieces
and reaches those
we know and respect,
it robs us of any vanity
and of the power to object.

*

My face is swollen from crying.
Someone brushes a damp strand of hair from my cheek.
I lie down inside my swollen face to cry.

The death of a loved one
remains the ugliest thing of all.

I yearn for the ugliest moments that had passed,
when there was still a chance to help her warm body.

Amid the cut flowers and medications,
I studied her hand.
Sometimes our eyes met, maybe
because I was sobbing without realizing it,
and once she uttered the only sentence
spoken that day: *khairat ast bachem?*

The sun shone in on us for so long,
we found ourselves sitting in the dark again.
The pump of her respirator measured the time we had left.

I yearn for the ugliest moments,
when I got to say goodbye to her cold body
four last times.

I yearn for the ugliest sounds
that our bodies, twisted with grief, emitted,
when pain still had a voice,
before it became a dull silence.

I was an animal, howling on all fours.
With every movement, an uncontrolled,
ugly wail escaped my body.

I was an animal, no room
for any human in my
ugly pain.

*

Bodies stand tightly packed in front of me,
behind me, beside me.
Like a swarm, together we cry and flee
on the heels of the casket.

Everyone around me is pale, dressed in black.
Everything I see is a blur; my eyes
are wet, I can no longer make out faces.
They all move to the right,
bow, rise,
pray, cry. I see
a black swarm
carrying her casket, and I imagine

it's the grief
that emerged from my body.
It's black and pale
and carrying my mother to her grave for me.

Why do we have to save face, even in death,
adorning the ground with flowers that cost more
than all her favorite dresses put together,
dresses that got to touch
her living body.

PALE

Death is so ugly,
but we dress it up
and give it a purpose,
a wreath,
a name.

At best we forget when looking at corpses
that they're corpses.
We lean in close to their faces.

Are we sure they're not just sleeping?

The final demonstration of respect for the dead
is translated quickly and easily into products
peddled to us in catalogues.
As we page through the binder, they ask:
How much did you love your mother?
Is she worth the 900-euro pine to you, or the 2,500-euro wild oak?

Families who opt for an open-casket funeral are opting
for a final display of the deceased. They are paying for one
final staging of the dead body, from the casket itself to the
elaborate preparation of the corpse. For open-casket services,
corpses are not only embalmed and generally readied, they
are also made-up.

Makeup is applied to the chilled body right before the funeral. A rich moisturizer seals the makeup and protects the dead face from parching. The body—which no longer moves, whose breast no longer rises and falls, no longer contains breath—simply lies there. A mortuary cosmetologist carefully places plastic wrap on the face. This helps the makeup set better. It also shields the deceased from any dust settling upon them. Though the dead may not move anymore, they are still present. Their bodies will collect dust like furniture, before they start to decompose like cadavers.

One cosmetologist, who works at a funeral home in Hollywood, explains that the deceased are done up according to a family's wishes, how they saw their loved one. They select reference photos for the makeup artist. If a woman elaborately styled her hair all her life, it's a final act of respect to lay her to rest with that hairdo. If the deceased had a mole with one long hair growing from it, one shows respect by allowing her to take it to the grave.

Nevertheless, the cosmetologist continues, some mortuary workers in the United States have their own take on how to prepare dead bodies. These approaches barely differ from what's pushed on living bodies. The living receive injections of Botox or hyaluronic acid to firm up their skin.

The dead, meanwhile, are injected with "feature filler," a chemical substance to plumpen and thus enliven the face.

Dead people look like dead people, and if they were sick before they died, they look like sick people who died. Some families, however, want the sunken features of the deceased filled and revived one last time, so they won't have to stare death in the face.

Embalmers give grandmothers the faces of mothers with their injections. They can make wrinkles disappear and a face look thirty years younger. The skin is padded, polished, colored. Often, though, discoloration that makes elderly or ill people appear elderly or ill will vanish on its own. As blood recedes from the skin and pallor sets in, some people's appearance almost seems improved in death. They look younger, less worn. If their skin tone is blue or translucent, a cosmetologist can help. Skin should not remind people of death's cold grip on the body, so morticians inject another chemical preservative manipulated with coloring agents. The cheeks now glow as though supplied with blood, and they are, in a sense—only it's formaldehyde. After all this, the dead appear alive and well when we bury and surrender them to decay.

*

Karl Rosenkranz, a nineteenth-century philosopher and student of Hegel's, writes in *Aesthetics of Ugliness* (1853) that fear of ghosts emerges from the contradictory notion that the dead could still be alive. It is not dead life that is eerie but the "thought of life in death."

Thanatology is the study of death and dying, a broad scientific field that encompasses all aspects of the physical phenomenon as well as its spiritual and social implications. Thanatopraxis, the many practices associated with thanatology, frequently involves beautifying the dead.

In Greek mythology, Thanatos is the god of the dead—one goal of thanatopraxis is the artificial delay of natural decomposition. Blood, fluids, and gases are released from the dead body through carefully placed incisions and replaced with a formaldehyde solution. The mortician closes the incisions, then washes the corpse and disinfects its orifices. Finally, the body is clothed, the hair styled, and makeup applied. The visual restoration of a corpse is especially involved when the individual suffered violence or illness in death. In Islam, it's forbidden.

All I know about these postmortem procedures comes from American TV and film, in scenes where the dead are put on display in open caskets for one last goodbye. This practice first emerged in Western cultures with the embalming of kings, the nobility, and Christian dignitaries, then spread to broader populations when the need arose to return soldiers to their families, or colonizers to their home countries, after they died.

The American Civil War was a turning point for the advance and popularization of embalming. The so-called

"American way of death" amounted to a cultural revolution, a democratizing shift in the presentation of bodies at life's end. No longer was it just kings and the canonized whose bodies were prepared for a final audience; as embalming grew more commercial, over time anyone could have access to it. This new market relied on industrialization and the emergence of chemical manufacturers, whose representatives swept across the land, pushing products and techniques. Funerals moved from the family home to professional undertakers, and the public preservation and presentation of the deceased became a primary component of the funeral business. More and more families started putting their dead on display, with businesses and other institutions helping them present the bodies at their best, most beautiful, most lifelike. Modern embalming practice thus moved away from medicine—from anatomical research and postmortem physical examinations—and formed its own profession: a profession with the single, great aesthetic goal of *putting on display.*

*

Mexican conceptual artist Teresa Margolles transforms bodies into images, works of art, to keep them from disintegrating and allow them to persist, though dead. Her work is not beautiful, but repellent, the bodies not embalmed, but fragmented, translated, concealed. Thomas Macho, an Austrian cultural philosopher, examines the work of Margolles in his 2007 essay "Ästhetik der Verwesung" (The Aesthetics of Decomposition). Macho introduces Margolles's art by explaining that, in some ways, the dead represent the "disgusting remains," the "last trace" of a process long concluded: "Dead bodies disintegrate, while pictures do not."

Margolles is not interested in *beautiful corpses*. She is drawn toward people who died a violent death. Though it is true that all humans die, that we all face death eventually, like the living, the dead are divided into rich and poor, beautiful and unbeautiful. Beautiful bodies are memorialized and laid to rest with dignity, whereas in Margolles's work, at times the dead are abandoned to mass graves, because they don't have anyone, or because their families were barred from providing even a simple burial. In 1999 Margolles exhibited a miscarried fetus contained within a block of cement. The mother, who was poor, had not wanted the hospital to dispose of the remains, so Margolles offered her a sort of entombment within conceptual artwork. In 2000 the artist created a piece around the severed, pierced tongue of a young murder victim who had suffered from addiction and whose mother could not afford his burial.

Margolles offered to cover the funeral fees if she could use the tongue in her piece—as a way to commemorate the many victims of their country's drug epidemic. The preserved tongue was thus wrested from silence, allowed to speak of the "squandering of an entire life," as Macho puts it. As for me, words fail.

I am still searching for words to describe the unfathomable ugliness of what was once the tongue of a living person being put on display for the art world. I don't find it ugly because it came from an ugly person, but because the desperation that compelled a mother to consent to having part of her son's body exhibited must be so hideous.

Is it Margolles's commentary on the capitalist art industry that's ugly, is it her art, the industry, or the dead bodies themselves? The answer is found in her somber aesthetic, which turns the mirror back on the questioner by translating the material remains of dead bodies into "erect plaster casts" or "traces of bodily fluids" on burial shrouds. She gathers the bodily traces of anonymous unhoused people and halts decay by chemically fixing the stains in the fabric, then presents them as paintings. It's the bloodied bedsheets or garments of deceased patients or children that lead me to suspect Margolles is obsessed with the corporeality of ugly deaths, an obsession that at times is more interested in the context of their deaths than in the dignity of the former bodies.

Is this work possible, its production acceptable, because— as Margolles contends—the people exhibited were demeaned and existed in ugly conditions all their lives? It's the waste products of the poor and ugly that ultimately end up in the artist's creations, only then they never *end*; then their dead bodies survive, translated into Margolles's language.

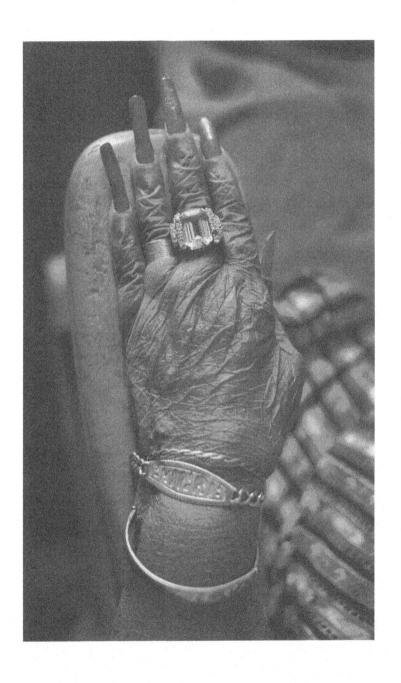

Margolles's interest extends beyond unbeautiful bodies to include unbeautiful fats. I read about her monochrome murals composed of body fat removed during liposuction. The exhibited fluids are anonymous, traces of bodies society viewed as a stain, until that is exactly what they became, just stains on fabric. These minimalist, documentary testimonies to unjust deaths, unbeautiful corpses, and scorned bodies do not diminish the ugliness or foulness of the corpses—on the contrary. Margolles's art touches and makes these qualities material before they have a chance to dissipate. She clings to the ugliest moment in other people's lives—the unfair end.

Thinking about her work, I find a response to my initial resistance from Margolles herself. In 2003 she said, "I work with inanimate bodies. . . . with that which rots." Then, as if taking the words out of my mouth, she asks, "How much does a dead body live through?"

DECOMPOSITION

*The first fright the deceased gives the living is that he doesn't
disappear, but rather stays.*

—**THOMAS MACHO**, "The Aesthetics of Decomposition"

A corpse exists on a threshold.
It passes from our bodies
into the materiality of the dead,
all the way to disintegration.
Before disintegrating, a reminder:
that could be us.

Julia Kristeva would say the corpse *horrifies* us.
We heave at the meaning it cleaves.

It is our body rebelling against death.
Corpses un-settle us.
Their absent presence shifts our settled self
outside our body.
For a second their chill passes over our skin
and we realize: if corpses exist,
so does our death.

The rejection of corpses is an act of distancing. We seek space between ourselves and the things we don't want, don't want to become, don't want to be.

The passage to decay begins in sick bodies, open wounds, injuries. We even sense our mortality in the feces we evacuate from our bodies, as though it weren't ours; we sense it in the waste we leave behind. What once nourished us now rots. Before long, what once propelled us now fails. And in our final moment, what remains is our body, naked and alone, when there's nothing left and everything turns to waste.

*

I don't want to look dead, but what I see in the mirror dismays me. I look dead. My skin is pale—not pale as fine china, pale as whiteness, or pale as Snow White, but pallid as a drowned body or patient in the intensive care unit in desperate need of a blood transfusion, or my own undead self hunting me down. Bags hang from my eyes, and my mouth is dry. In the cabinet is some blood-red lipstick, which I draw across my lips. I dab my fingers in the pigment, then blend it into my cheeks to incorporate the color into my complexion. I want to look ruddy, alive and well. When I put on makeup, I want it to look like I'm alive.

V. RECONCILIATION

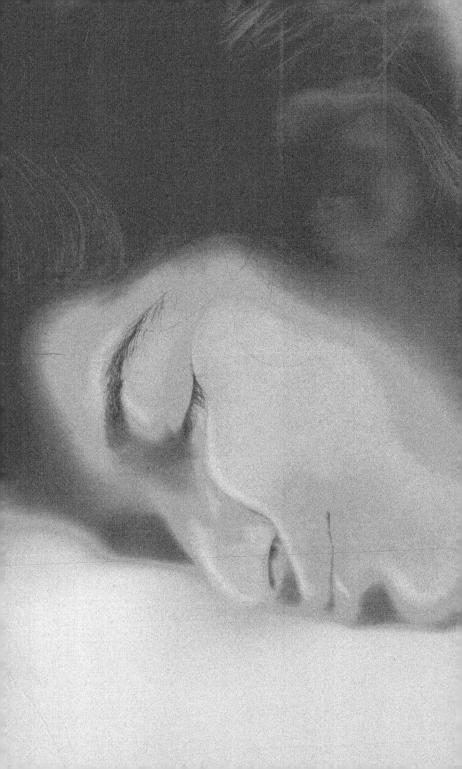

Where is the Ugly in you? What is it trying to teach you?

—MIA MINGUS, "Moving Toward the Ugly:
A Politic Beyond Desirability"

At this point, after all the images projected onto our bodies we've gone through to get here, we have to ask: What do we do with this information? Why endure the painful memory of moments of self-loathing, disgust, humiliation? Why look so intently at ugliness and self-estrangement—to what end? What can be done with the idea of ugliness, now that we're perhaps better able to grasp it? This final chapter is titled "Reconciliation." The reconciliation I hope to find would dismantle the destructive dichotomy that has defined everything up till now: beauty or normality insisting on ugliness as its foil. Reconciliation means abolishing this antagonism by means of connection and understanding—until bodies are permitted to be just bodies and pictures can no longer cut through skin.

*

The classic aesthetic of the West extends far beyond Europe and the United States, yet is geared exclusively toward the cultural legacy and elite bodies of those places. It is dualistic, antagonistic, and requires its antithesis at all times: everything within this aesthetic develops in contrast to the Other.

Just as Hazaras are referred to in polemical texts as ugly crea-
tures, as rebellious people who eat rats and insects, so were the
demons in the Shahnama . . . So I started painting the demon as
a collective portrait of my ancestors and my own self.

—KHADIM ALI, "Demons of Otherness"

Ugliness is embedded in a history of colonialism and dehumanization. How can we learn from those who have been
marginalized in this way? How have groups that in many
cases continue to suffer from these labels responded, survived, or resisted? The artist Khadim Ali—who belongs to
the Hazara community, a historically persecuted minority
from Afghanistan—has discussed how he reclaims and reap-
propriates the ugly imagery and demonic roles assigned to his
ancestors in regional Farsi literature. The American painter
Kerry James Marshall reimagines Black love, joy, and everyday life in works that combine elements of Western art history with a hyperbolic use of black-hued paint as the skin
color of his subjects. What was weaponized against Black
people, turns into the iconic aesthetic of his art.

Julia Kristeva's essay "Powers of Horror" further elucidates
the notion of absolute rejection, asking if there is something
evolutionary, deeply biological about the fact that we cannot

stand a certain sight, smell, or Other? The way our bodies react to spoiled milk or a cadaver signals something to us. Kristeva writes that it is "not lack of cleanliness or health that causes abjection but what disturbs identity, system, order"—essentially, that which blurs the line between the self and the Other. Abjection arises from a disruption to our sense of normality. This reaction to ambiguity or transgression is not innate but socially constructed, reinforcing societal norms and boundaries. Historically this power of horror has been effectively weaponized against what was foreign, new, or antagonized.

Walter Mignolo and Rolando Vázquez, in their article "Decolonial AestheSis: Colonial Wounds/Decolonial Healings," critique Immanuel Kant's formalization of aesthetics, which established rules for perception and sensing, favoring Eurocentric tenets of beauty. They draw a critical distinction between "aestheTics," the formalized, doctrinal theory of beauty, and "aestheSis," the innate capacity to sense and perceive inherent in all humans, if not most beings. AestheTics, they argue, has historically acted as a colonizer of sensory experience, imposing hierarchical structures on what is deemed beautiful, how to formally judge and intellectualize the sensual world, and conversely, what or who is deemed ugly.

Mignolo and Vázquez argue that aesthetics, as a normative force, has reduced sensory experience to discrete, objectifiable categories, much like the Western educational system has done to the process of learning. This reductionist view not only marginalizes non-normative sensory experiences but also reinforces colonial power structures. By recognizing the historical and contextual origins of terms like aesthetics, they contend, we can dismantle their claims to universality and truth.

Kristeva's analysis aligns with Mignolo and Vázquez's critique, suggesting that the fear and rejection of the Other—often labeled as ugly—is a product of societal learning rather than an objective reality. Like aesthetics and abjection, ugliness, in this reframing, is revealed not as an inherent quality but as a constructed idea within a very specific context. If it's *just* an idea, we might also be in the position to *simply* unlearn it, to ultimately reject it. The insight challenges the perception of ugliness as a timeless, universal concept. Instead, it is a dynamic social construct, essentially an empty one, laden with meaning and perpetuated by the collective social body to maintain order, identity, and power.

*

They were meant to be pictures that captured me on days I wanted to be seen. I had already finished writing this book when D. sent me the press photos. I could have sworn I was beaming in them; my memory of those photographed days was of how lovely and full they were.

What I find myself looking at instead casts doubt on those warm memories. My sad face looks back at me: my skin is dirty, dry, orange. My photographed eyes are tired and throw me back to the start of this book, back to my beginnings—fourteen ugly mugs at fourteen years old. Have I not learned anything? After all I've written about ugliness for this book, all it takes is the impression of having aged unawares to send me back to square one?

My mother always said faces were fleeting. What she meant was beauty.

How could my face fade on me like that, after I worked so hard getting to know and love it? No sooner do I learn to love this face than it changes. I kept myself waiting for so long, my face got me back for it by aging.

An ocean of observations lies between ugliness and these photos, D. writes back, after I tell him his pictures tested my book's stated objectives. His point is greater than he might realize, as it also reminds me: I wish to become reconciled with myself, and reconciliation is found beyond the realm of dichotomy. I wish to learn to see and be seen without the chagrin of a person who fears proximity to ugliness. Without the chagrin of a person who feels they must love every shadow they cast.

VISUAL INJUSTICE

As a kid, I knew that monsters were far more gentle and more desirable than the monsters living inside "nice people."... And I think accepting that you are a monster gives you the leeway to not behave like one. When you deny being a monster, you behave like one.

—GUILLERMO DEL TORO

In *Ugliness: A Cultural History*, Henderson writes that, unlike some, she did not aim to compile a sensational catalogue of the marginalized and marked, also known as the ugly. Instead, she wanted to create an overview of related terms and cultural practices that have arisen around ugly groups, everything from exploitation and extermination to "fixing" and even eroticizing. Though it might at first glance seem to be an account of disjointed cases, when taken together, these examples suggest patterns and connections. Henderson's work thus collects social processes that produce ugliness and does not simply collate documents about *the ugly*. The question guiding her is not "Who are the ugly?" but rather, "How does ugliness come into being?" By contrast, Umberto Eco's own book *On Ugliness* reads like a treatise in which the ugly are mostly mute. The violence they have endured is reproduced uncritically as if in a cabinet of curiosities, and ultimately, their ugliness is simply left untouched, unchallenged.

Learning to set aside the ugliness in our gaze does not mean ugliness will cease to exist. When we start rejecting ugliness as a concept and replacing it in speech with euphemisms, coded adjectives, or air quotes, the experienced material reality of the so-called ugly remains largely unchanged. Really, when we hunt for ugliness in ourselves, it isn't necessarily that we hate our pudgy thighs, dirty hands, hairy belly, or hunched back; it's that we fear the categorical proximity to those our society hates. We try to maintain distance between ourselves and anything that could be deemed unproductive, indigent, animal, or inept—any and all counterpoints to our modern ideas of how humans should be or behave. The ugly don't exist because they are ugly, but because they endure ugliness. In this case, ugliness is the hate-based exclusion found in the judgment and behaviors of others. It is expressed through various forms of sensory rejection, especially visual: we experience this ugliness in our self-image as well as in how the Other sees us and how we see the Other. It can mean a rejection of the self as readily as that of the Other, but either way, the act is connected to the repudiation of deviance, variation, and perceived indolence—a rejection of anything that does not feed (or that disturbs) the growth and order of modern society. Ugliness is a tool used against those for whom the system has no desired use other than rejection.

*

In 1898 the Barnum & Bailey Circus—whose founder, P. T. Barnum, we met earlier—began a residency in London as part of a four-year European tour. At the time, the world-famous show employed forty professional "human curiosities," the largest troupe of sideshow artists in history. In *Staging Stigma*, Michael M. Chemers cites a London newspaper that on January 6, 1899, reported a "revolt of the freaks"—one of the first-ever instances of self-organization among American performers. The "freaks" were not "revolting" over working conditions, however, but instead fighting for "semantic principles [and] linguistic dignity." The paper reported on a clandestine meeting called by Annie Jones, a *bearded lady*. At the gathering, Jones delivered a speech on the term *freak* and why its use should be halted. Attendees signed the resolution she had drafted opposing the word, an "indignity" that had been applied to the undersigned sometimes with, sometimes without consent. The document emphasizes that the performers' "certain marked and distinctive characteristics of mind and body" were no reason to classify them as "freaks." In closing, the collective declared that "in the opinion of many, some of us are . . . superior persons . . . with extraordinary attributes." The resolution called for a general strike and thus for a collective refusal to work until those responsible for the show and its marketing dropped the term and eliminated its traces. The signatories chose a new term for themselves—*prodigies*—and with it, a narrative that construed their unique qualities as superiority, rather than deviation.

*

In *The Ugly Laws: Disability in Public* (2009), Susan M. Schweik writes about nineteenth-century ordinances against "ugliness" in the United States and Europe, which barred individuals deemed unattractive or disturbing from certain public spaces. Their bodies sullied the aspect of such sites, the laws stated, as they were *poor, deformed, diseased,* or otherwise *unsightly.* They should not be permitted to disturb beautiful, normal people in their visual experience of public spaces. A pretty young lady of means taking the air in the park or a well-situated family making their way home should not be subjected to discomfiture at the sight of a beggar or otherwise vexatious figure.

Ugly laws reveal a segregation line undergirding everything from ugliness to unlawful detention: Who has the right to be seen by whom? In many places today, similar restrictions and private business bans apply to poor or unhoused people, with discipline enforced by police. Even at the entrance to a nightclub, prejudice regarding physical attractiveness, guest "comfort," and belonging reigns supreme. Nineteenth-century ugly laws led to increased public presence of police, deployed to safeguard the interests and comfort of the white middle class against the alleged threat that discriminated groups—the losers—posed within the same society. Schweik connects this development to industrialization and the desire for *beautiful spaces*, where one could escape the ugly sight of industrial exploitation and misery in one's home nation, now no longer relegated to the colonies. She describes ugly laws as just one structural means of culling ugliness, others including immigration laws, sterilization, and eugenics. The unsightly were not only barred from certain spaces, they were confined to others created just for them, like prisons or psychiatric clinics. Refugee camps can be viewed within the same category, as they serve to restrict the movement of people who supposedly pose a threat to national harmony.

*

The feminist sociologists Ela Przybylo and Sara Rodrigues refuse to reduce ugliness to the empirical qualities of bodies, spaces, or things. Instead, they maintain that ugliness serves a *social* function by upholding societal notions of value and entitlement: Whose life is more worth living? Who gets to make demands of life? As editors of the reader *On the Politics of Ugliness*, Przybylo and Rodrigues attempt to translate the politicization of ugliness into new ways of seeing and being seen that would allow a person to possess "ugly" features without denigration. Following this premise, they dive deep into the material and political consequences of ugliness, the "unjust distribution of wealth and power" based on one's grouping by external characteristics. Such denigration, the editors suggest, amounts to "visual injustice."

*

In *Belly of the Beast: The Politics of Anti-Fatness as Anti-Blackness*, Da'Shaun L. Harrison questions why we would equate insecurity with "personal and moral failing" when it's actually the result of domination. They write, "If the politicization of Ugly leads to the social, political, economic, and physical death of a person, they are bound to feel unprotected, uncared for, and unconfident." The insecurity experienced by people marked as ugly, Harrison continues, is not only justified—the logical outcome of lived reality—it is itself a political feeling that emerges from one's personal circumstances, whose creation is also political. Whether a repudiated body is insecure or self-confident does not alter the material reality of its repudiation. For that reason, Harrison believes that the perception and assumption of one's own perpetual insecurity "better [contextualizes]" the reality of hated bodies: "You can't beat people down forever and expect that they never feel the effects of that continued beating."

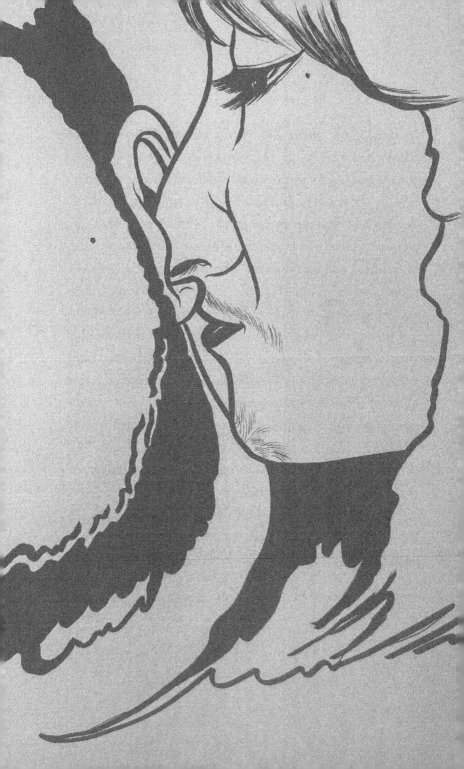

NEGATED BEAUTY

my beauty is so tremendous
they had me believe so long it was not there—
so when i finally found it, here:
in all of the places i was taught to hate

    —ALOK, "My Beauty is Tremendous"

Mia Mingus delivered the keynote address at the 2011 Femmes of Color Symposium in Oakland about the feminist need to rethink ugliness. I first read the speech, titled "Moving Toward the Ugly: A Politic Beyond Desirability," on the activist's blog many years later, after stumbling across a conversation between Mingus and the writer, performance artist, and activist ALOK. My encounter with her plea for more ugliness shook me in every sense. Until that point, I had sought a way into the realm of beauty. I thought I could recruit ethical arguments and aesthetic drawings to earn this access; I thought I might convince others, and maybe even myself, that I'm beautiful too.

Mingus, however, dispenses with the concept of beauty entirely. She writes:

> We must shift from a politic of desirability and beauty to a politic of ugly and magnificence. That

moves us closer to bodies and movements that disrupt, dismantle, disturb. Bodies and movements ready to throw down and create a different way *for all of us, not just some of us.*

Not just some of us . . . these final words rattled me. They introduced me to a new sense of shame—not the shame of being seen as *ugly*, but of being thought *beautiful* and thus joining the side of injustice. Mingus sees so much violence and exclusion in the idea of beauty that she suggests an alternate guiding vision: *magnificence.* One is not born magnificent, based on appearance, but rather becomes magnificent through experience. Mingus defines the magnificent body primarily as a disabled body, one that lives with disability; this body is impressive in its disability, not in spite of it, in its capacity for resilience, endurance, survival. Though Mingus's personal experience with ableism is grounded in disability and queerness, she views the notion of having to be *able* within the system as emblematic of all forms of exclusion.

On our quest for beauty, *what do we do with bodies that can't change?* Mingus does not want to chase after something that rejects her and her body: "There is only the illusion of solace in beauty." Even those bodies that might well attain beauty cannot expect to find permanent, unconditional power there.

In the aging, illness, and infirmity that every body encounters, we all come to recognize how unreliable and ultimately unfaithful beauty is; it will forsake us. Ugliness holds a different kind of assurance. Mingus therefore attributes all manner of magnificence to ugliness, whereas beauty is meager, exclusive, and fleeting. She implores us "to not be afraid of the Ugly—in each other or ourselves." We must also learn to respect the ugly, because it will show us how we don't want to make other people feel. If given the choice, we should side against the gawkers and with the ugly.

We were taught that the only lives that are worthwhile are those that are beautiful. Only those whom others envy possess something worth having. In her conversation with ALOK, Mingus explains that ugliness teaches us intimacy and trust through vulnerability. "In order to be vulnerable, you have to reveal parts of yourself that are dismissed as capital-U Ugly" and that may lead to interdependence. Mingus's own disability has shown her how "inescapable" interdependence can produce deep relationships and meaningful community, provided the others do not fear and flee ugliness. Disability has a tangible quality that does not allow people to look the other way or belie ugliness, she says. Her call to respect ugliness does not mean everyone should abandon the search for beauty, just because she has; instead, those searching for it should question its objectives and criteria: "When we feel validated, what are we actually feeling validated by?"

*

I, too, am beautiful.

I, too, am ugly.

On my search for beauty in those places I had so long associated with shame and hatred, I happened upon ugliness. I knew it well from personal experience or seeing it in others, but I decided to reacquaint myself with ugliness, to get to know its history and many facets obscured by humanity. On my search for beauty in a curved nose or a lady's thick beard, I learned about the violence this beauty has engendered and the damaged lives it has on its conscience. Finally, I learned to respect ugliness: as an enduring reflection, not just of myself in the mirror, but of our humanness. Ugliness alone reflects a truth that transcends images and words in bearing witness to the vulnerability of human life and the organic limits of the many abstract, general ideals imposed on us. I must respect ugliness as a witness, archive, test, and reflection before I can return to my search for other, negated beauties.

The more I learn about ugliness, the more I become reconciled to it. I fear it less and less, even as a certain reverence remains. Ugliness is anything but skin-deep. It engages us at an existential level, questioning the meaning and value of our lives. When we become reconciled to ugliness, it opens the door to Mingus's notion of magnificence, this other value that takes its shape from our existence, not from a utility to others or conformity to those we are forced to be.

I am ugly, because I am.
I am beautiful, because I am.

When we dismantle the dichotomy of beauty and ugliness, the conflict between the two subsides within us too. We are ugly and beautiful, by turns and at once.

Several years ago, when I started drawing self-portraits, I tried to employ the aestheticizing gaze of an artist to reconcile myself to my ugliness. I hoped that, by looking at forms, lines, and planes like a professional, I would tap into a different way of understanding and working with them, beyond obtuse vanity. Conceiving of my nose as a sculpture, my face as a canvas, and my hair as drawn lines left no space for the poles of ugly and beautiful. Aestheticizing my shameful features—translating them into a visual language—allowed me to start inching away from my fear of ugliness.

Negated beauty was my attempt to see my rejected body differently, to confront it and thus insert myself anew into my body and image of myself. While it might be easy to create a beautiful representation of an ugly thing and thus unsettle the contradiction (art can do that, find a language beyond dichotomies), negated beauty is ultimately an aesthetic response to a physical question. This response is not without its limitations, of course, day-to-day reality being more complex and mutable than questions of visual representation. On my search for beauty, it was negated beauty that led me to places I could make my own. The reconciliation with ugliness will, however, keep challenging me. I will have to demand it of myself every day, remind myself every day, admonish my gaze, and defy my fear and disgust. I cannot reconcile myself to ugliness through aesthetics and verse alone. Reconciliation requires more of me, namely acknowledging my humanity and mortality—and with them, the unpredictable, ambiguous, and ever-challenging material reality in which we all live.

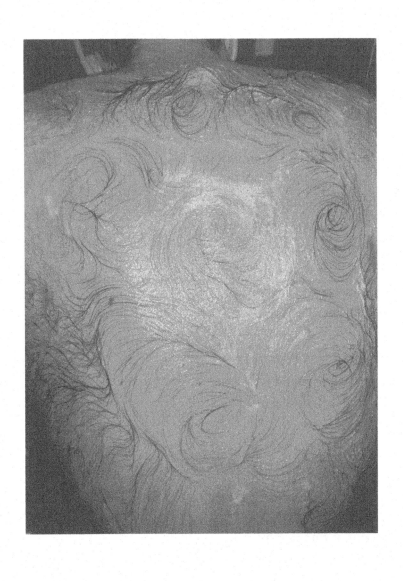

In the shadow of my nose is a garden.
A garden where black grass grows
and faces resemble landscapes.

From the south, two eyebrows,
the nose rising between them,
giving comfort to the thoughts.
Black hair frames the upper lip,
grows up the forearms
and under the sleeves.

Hands swim in the water.
In the reflection I see
a profile like a sickle
and reach for it

slicing gaping wounds in all your glances.
And there, just where the pain makes you stop and think,
that's the very place
I put down my roots.

Hatched lines like black badges
rise in sharp relief,
turning away from whiteness.
Every hair, every stroke, every line
unwanted war paint.
Though they would have been soft and gentle
if touched
by a conciliatory hand.

What a waste, every time
the black hair
collects in the drain.
What resistance,
every time it rises again
to confront the blade.
In the shadow of my nose is a place
where difference is free
to eclipse conformity;

where the I in place of nothing,
will have uncovered
our gaze and yours.

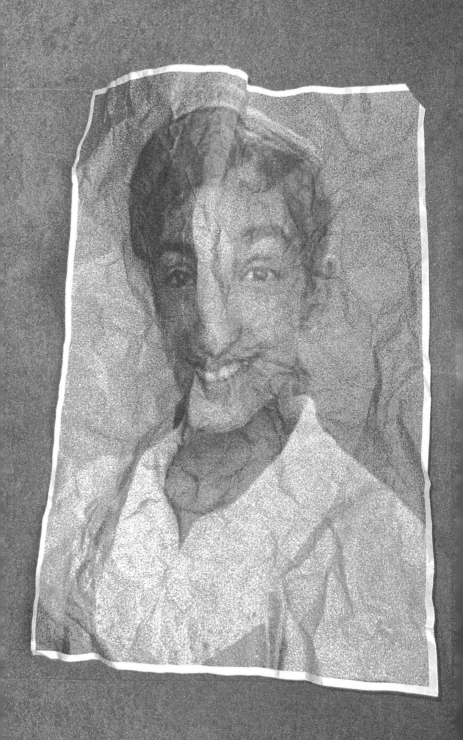

WORKS CITED

Works cited in order they appear in text (with chapter titles)

HATRED

Pressler, Jessica. "Maybe She Had So Much Money She Just Lost Track of It." *New York Magazine*, May 28, 2018. https://jessicapressler.com/maybe-she-had-so-much-money-she-just-lost-track-of-it/1207.

Fanon, Frantz. *Black Skin, White Masks*. Translated by Charles Lam Markmann. London: Pluto Press, 2008.

———. *Toward the African Revolution*. Translated by Haakon Chevalier. New York: Grove Press, 1969.

NASAL ANALYSIS

Gilman, Sander L. *Making the Body Beautiful: A Cultural History of Aesthetic Surgery*. Princeton: Princeton University Press, 2000.

Lin, Ji. "Chinese Man Sues Wife after 'Ugly' Baby Born." *The Irish Examiner*, October 31, 2012. https://www.irishexaminer.com/news/arid-20212463.html.

Galton, Francis. "Generic Images." *Nineteenth Century* 6 (July 1879): 157–69. https://galton.org/essays/1870-1879/galton-1879-generic-images.pdf.

———. "Composite Portraits, Made by Combining Those of Many Different Persons into a Single Resultant Figure." *Nature* 18 (May 1878): 97–100. https://galton.org/essays/1870-1879/galton-1878-nature-composite.pdf.

Belden-Adams, Kris. *Eugenics, "Aristogenics," Photography: Picturing Privilege*. New York: Routledge, 2020.

Maxwell, Anne. *Picture Imperfect: Photography and Eugenics, 1879-1940*. Liverpool: Liverpool University Press, 2008.

Gilman, Sander L. *Seeing the Insane: A Visual and Cultural History of Our Attitudes Toward the Mentally Ill*. Brattleboro, VT: Echo Point Books & Media, 2014.

Lavater, Johann Caspar. *Essays on Physiognomy, Calculated to Extend the Knowledge and the Love of Mankind*. Translated by C. Moore. London: H. D. Symonds, 1797.

Gray, Richard T. *About Face: German Physiognomic Thought from Lavater to Auschwitz*. Detroit: Wayne State University Press, 2004.

Zeitler, Annika. "Human Zoos: When People Were the Exhibits." *Deutsche Welle*, March 10, 2017. https://www.dw.com/en/human-zoos-when-people-were-the-exhibits/a-37748193.

Harrisburg University of Science and Technology. "HU Facial Recognition Software Predicts Criminality," May 5, 2020. https://web.archive.org/web/20200506013352/https:/harrisburgu.edu/hu-facial-recognition-software-identifies-potential-criminals.

Coalition for Critical Technology. "Abolish the #TechToPrisonPipeline," June 23, 2020. https://medium.com/@CoalitionForCriticalTechnology/abolish-the-techtoprisonpipeline-9b5b14366b16.

Dieffenbach, Johann Friedrich. *Der Aether gegen den Schmerz*. Berlin: A. Hirschwald, 1847.

Celletti, Erin Nicole. "The Complete Guide to Rhinoplasty." *Allure*, May 15, 2018. https://www.allure.com/story/rhinoplasty-everything-you-need-to-know.

Schadow, Johann Gottfried. *National-Physiognomien oder Beobachtungen über den Unterschied der Gesichtszüge und der äußeren Gestalt des Körpers*, 1835.

Rady Rahban, MD. "Ethnic Rhinoplasty," accessed May 14, 2024. https://www.radyrahban.com/procedures/nose/ethnic-rhinoplasty.php.

Franklyn, Sofia. "The Brutal Truth About Plastic Surgery with Dr. Rady Rahban." March 9, 2023. YouTube video, 1:22:27. https://www.youtube.com/watch?v=orFDXcjAZbU.

Brücke, Ernst. *The Human Figure: Its Beauties and Defects*. London: H. Grevel & Co., 1900.

Gazagnadou, Didier. "Diffusion of Cultural Models, Body Transformations and Technology in Iran: Iranian Women and Cosmetic Nose Surgery." *Anthropology of the Middle East* 1, no. 1 (Spring 2006): 106–11. https://doi.org/10.3167/ame.2006.010108.

Bourdieu, Pierre. *Distinction: A Social Critique of the Judgement of Taste*. Translated by Richard Nice. Cambridge, MA: Harvard University Press, 1987.

Lenehan, Sara. "Nose Aesthetics: Rhinoplasty and Identity in Tehran." *Anthropology of the Middle East* 6, no. 1 (Spring 2011): 47–62. https://doi.org/10.3167/ame.2011.060105.

Rahbari, Ladan, Susan Dierickx, Chia Longman, and Gily Coene. "'Kill Me but Make Me Beautiful': Harm and Agency in Female Beauty Practices in Contemporary Iran." *Iran & the Caucasus* 22, no. 1 (2018): 50–60.

Harper's Bazaar. "Bella Hadid's Face Measured for Physical Perfection by a Harley Street Surgeon." October 15, 2019. https://www.harpersbazaar.com/uk/beauty/a29469684/bella-hadid-most-beautiful-woman.

Haskell, Rob. "Bella From the Heart: On Health Struggles, Happiness, and Everything in Between." *Vogue*, March 15, 2022. https://www.vogue.com/article/bella-hadid-cover-april-2022.

Kim Kardashian (@KimKardashian), "I said you will see when I have kids, they will have the same nose as me." Twitter, February 13, 2019, 5:03 p.m. https://twitter.com/kimkardashian/status/1095805720774115329.

Entertainment Tonight!, "Kylie Jenner Wishes She'd NEVER Gotten Any Cosmetic Work Done," YouTube Video, 0:07, April 27, 2023. https://www.youtube.com/watch?v=DPvcTzCTknk.

Jenner, Kylie. "Kontrol." Interview by Nicolaia Rips. *HommeGirls*, May 2023. https://www.hommegirls.com/blogs/volume-9/kontrol.

Widdows, Heather. *Perfect Me: Beauty as an Ethical Ideal.* Princeton: Princeton University Press, 2018.

Tolentino, Jia. "The Age of Instagram Face: How Social Media, FaceTune, and Plastic Surgery Created a Single, Cyborgian Look." *The New Yorker*, December 12, 2019. https://www.newyorker.com/culture/decade-in-review/the-age-of-instagram-face.

Benjamin, Walter. "The Work of Art in the Age of Mechanical Reproduction." In *Illuminations*, edited by Hannah Arendt, translated by Harry Zohn. New York: Schocken Books, 1969.

WOLF-GIRL

White, Richard Grant. *The Fall of Man: Or, The Loves of the Gorillas.* New York: G. W. Carleton & Co., 1871.

Darwin, Charles. *The Descent of Man, and Selection in Relation to Sex.* London: John Murray, 1871.

McCafferty, Lawrence K. "Hypertrichosis and Its Treatment." *New York Medical Journal*, December 5, 2023.

Herzig, Rebecca M. *Plucked: A History of Hair Removal.* New York: New York University Press, 2015.

Goodall, Jane R. *Performance and Evolution in the Age of Darwin: Out of the Natural Order*. London: Routledge, 2002.

Henderson, Gretchen E. *Ugliness: A Cultural History*. Chicago: University of Chicago Press, 2015.

Chemers, Michael M. *Staging Stigma: A Critical Examination of the American Freak Show*. New York: Palgrave Macmillan, 2008.

Garland-Thomson, Rosemarie. "Making Freaks: Visual Rhetorics and the Spectacle of Julia Pastrana." In *Thinking the Limits of the Body*, edited by Jeffrey Jerome Cohen and Gail Weiss, 129–44. Albany: State University of New York Press, 2003.

Norwegian National Committee for the Evaluation of Research on Human Remains. "Statement Concerning the Remains of Julia Pastrana." De nasjonale forskningsetiske komiteene, June 6, 2012. https://www.forskningsetikk.no/om-oss/komiteer-og-utvalg/skjelettutvalget/uttalelser/statement-concerning-the-remains-of-julia-pastrana.

Lyons, Harriet, and Rebecca Rosenblatt. "Body Hair: The Last Frontier." *Ms.*, July 1, 1972.

Mermin, Liz, dir. *The Beauty Academy of Kabul*. 2004; Magic Lantern Media Inc., 2005. Film.

Nguyen, Mimi Thi. "The Biopower of Beauty: Humanitarian Imperialisms and Global Feminisms in an Age of Terror." *Signs* 36, no. 2 (Winter 2011): 359–83. https://doi.org/10.1086/655914.

Billaud, Julie. *Kabul Carnival: Gender Politics in Postwar Afghanistan*. Philadelphia: University of Pennsylvania Press, 2015.

THE UNDEAD

Brenez, Nicole. "Women in Window: *The House Is Black* by Forugh

Farrokhzad." Translated by Eunjung Joo. *Sabzian*, December 15, 2021. https://www.sabzian.be/text/women-in-window.

Sontag, Susan. *Illness as Metaphor.* New York: Farrar, Straus and Giroux, 1977.

Remoundakis, Epaminondas, and Maurice Born. *Vies et morts d'un Crétois lépreux. Suivi de Archéologie d'une arrogance.* Toulouse, Marseille: Anacharsis, 2015.

Rosenkranz, Karl. *Aesthetics of Ugliness.* Translated by Andrei Pop and Mechtild Widrich. London: Bloomsbury Academic, 2015.

Macho, Thomas. "Die Ästhetik Der Verwesung." In *Die neue Sichtbarkeit des Todes*, edited by Thomas Macho and Kristin Marek. Leiden: Brill, 2007.

Kristeva, Julia. *Powers of Horror: An Essay on Abjection.* Translated by Leon S. Roudiez. New York: Columbia University Press, 1982.

RECONCILIATION

Mingus, Mia. "Moving Toward the Ugly: A Politic Beyond Desirability." Keynote speech at Femmes of Color Symposium, Oakland, CA, August 21, 2011. https://leavingevidence.wordpress.com/2011/08/22/moving-toward-the-ugly-a-politic-beyond-desirability.

Ali, Khadim. "Demons of Otherness." Interview by Safdar Ahmed. *Sydney Review of Books*, November 22, 2021. https://sydneyreviewofbooks.com/interview/demons-of-otherness-khadim-ali.

Mignolo, Walter, and Rolando Vázquez. "Decolonial AestheSis: Colonial Wounds/Decolonial Healings." *Social Text*, July 15, 2013. https://socialtextjournal.org/periscope_article/decolonial-aesthesis-colonial-woundsdecolonial-healings.

Applebaum, Stephen. "Guillermo del Toro on the Deeper Meaning in *The*

Shape of Water." *The National News*, March 5, 2018. https://www.thenational news.com/arts-culture/film/guillermo-del-toro-on-the-deeper-meaning-in-the-shape-of-water-1.699621.

Eco, Umberto. *On Ugliness.* New York: Rizzoli, 2011.

Schweik, Susan M. *The Ugly Laws: Disability in Public.* New York: New York University Press, 2009.

Rodrigues, Sara, and Ela Przybylo, eds. *On the Politics of Ugliness.* London: Palgrave Macmillan, 2018.

Harrison, Da'Shaun L. *Belly of the Beast: The Politics of Anti-Fatness as Anti-Blackness.* Berkeley: North Atlantic Books, 2021.

ALOK. "MY BEAUTY IS TREMENDOUS." *ALOK*, July 4, 2019. https:// www.alokvmenon.com/blog/2019/7/5/my-beauty-is-tremendous.

Mingus, Mia. "Why Ugliness Is Vital in the Age of Social Media." Interview by ALOK. *Them*, October 26, 2018. https://www.them.us/story/ugliness-disability-mia-mingus.

ILLUSTRATION CREDITS

116 Charles Darwin (*A Venerable Orang-Outang. A Contribution to Unnatural History*) published by/after Frederick Arnold; Unknown artist © National Portrait Gallery, London

126 © Moshtari Hilal

132/133 © Moshtari Hilal: *Zwei Arme/Two Arms*, 2023

138 Film still © Yumna al-Arashi: *Shedding Skin*, Film, 2017

141 Collage © Moshtari Hilal, using images from *Everywoman—Latvian Dads and Kabul Beauty Salon*, Al Jazeera English. https://www.youtube.com/watch?v=MXFCeVrP588, 28.08.2007, accessed May 2023.

144 © Forough Alaei: *Crying for Freedom*, 2019

152 Film still from *The House is Black* (Forugh Farrokhzad, 1963) © Fondazione Cineteca di Bologna, restored by Fondazione Cineteca di Bologna and Ecran Noir productions in collaboration with Ebrahim Golestan.

177 © Robert van der Hilst: "Africa," photo taken in Havana, 1987.

180 © Moshtari Hilal: *Selbstbetrachtung/Self Reflection*, 2023

192 © Moshtari Hilal: *Nasal Analysis*

199 Mona Hatoum: *Van Gogh's Back*, 1995 © Mona Hatoum 2024. Courtesy the artist

202 © Moshtari Hilal: "Crumpled Paper"

MOSHTARI HILAL is a visual artist, writer, and curator based in Hamburg and Berlin. Born in Afghanistan, she studied Islamic studies and political science in Hamburg, Berlin, and London.

ELISABETH LAUFFER is the recipient of the 2014 Gutekunst Translation Prize. After graduating from Wesleyan University, she lived in Berlin and has a master's in education from Harvard.

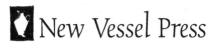New Vessel Press

For more information, please visit
newvesselpress.com.